Documentation for Athletic Training

Documentation
for Athletic
Training

Jeff G. Konin, PhD, ATC, PT

Assistant Athletic Director for Sports Medicine
Assistant Professor of Health Sciences
Clinical Coordinator of Athletic Training
James Madison University
Harrisonburg, Virginia

Margaret A. Frederick, MS, ATC

Instructor and Coordinator of Clinical Education
Longwood University
Farmville, Virginia

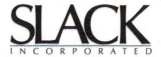

An innovative information, education, and management company
6900 Grove Road • Thorofare, NJ 08086

ISBN: 978-1-55642-641-4

The work SLACK Incorporated publishes is peer reviewed. Prior to publication, recognized leaders in the field, educators, and clinicians provide important feedback on the concept and content that we publish. We welcome feedback on this work.

Printed in the United States of America.

Library of Congress Cataloging-in-Publication Data
Konin, Jeff G.
  Documentation for athletic training / Jeff G. Konin, Meg Frederick.
     p. ; cm.
  Includes bibliographical references and index.
  ISBN-13: 978-1-55642-641-4 (alk. paper)
  ISBN-10: 1-55642-641-0 (alk. paper)
1. Physical education and training--Documentation. 2. Athletes--Training of--Documentation. I. Frederick, Meg. II. Title.

GV207.4.K66 2005
613.7--dc22

                                        2004023830

Published by: SLACK Incorporated
                 6900 Grove Road
                 Thorofare, NJ 08086 USA
                 Telephone: 856-848-1000
                 Fax: 856-853-5991
                 www.slackbooks.com

Contact SLACK Incorporated for more information about other books in this field or about the availability of our books from distributors outside the United States.

Last digit is print number: 10   9   8   7   6   5   4   3   2

DEDICATION

To all the athletic training students who are entering a world of information whereby the lack of proper documentation will be the demise of those who serve good will. To KJ and Christopher, whose elementary school writing skills are already better than their dad's!
JGK

To my parents, Peggy and Larry, for always showing me the way.
To Robert, for your love, your laughter, your strength, and your support. I love you always.
MAF

CONTENTS

Acknowledgments

Many individuals have contributed to the development of this book in one way or another. Some of our very first mentors in the profession, Dr. Herb Amato, Dr. Malissa Martin, Leah Gutekunst, Dr. Dave Yeo, Dr. Dave Perrin, and Lance Fujiwara, have been influential in our careers and helped to establish the foundation for our earliest forms of writing. As always, the wonderful people at SLACK Incorporated played a large role in seeing this project to fruition: John Bond, Amy McShane, Lauren Plummer, Michelle Gatt, Jessica Sycz, and especially Carrie Kotlar. Without this fine group of individuals who represent an amazing publishing company, we would not have been able to produce yet another academic contribution to the profession of athletic training. Thanks to the many generous certified athletic trainers who were kind enough to allow us to use their documents and forms as part of our appendices. The meat of the book lies in the labor of the contributors. To Todd Babcock, Nikki Beil, Dan Campbell, Mike Fahrner, Tamerah Hunt, John Kaltenborn, Karen Lew, and Sheila Nicholson, to whom we owe a great deal of gratitude, we say THANK YOU!

Jeff G. Konin
Margaret A. Frederick

ABOUT THE AUTHORS

Jeff G. Konin, PhD, ATC, PT, serves as the Assistant Athletic Director for Sports Medicine and as an Assistant Professor in the Department of Health Sciences at James Madison University. He received his undergraduate degree in Physical Education in 1988 from Eastern Connecticut State University, a Master of Education in Athletic Training/Sports Medicine from the University of Virginia in 1989, and a Master of Physical Therapy from the University of Delaware in 1994. He earned his PhD in Physical Therapy from Nova Southeastern University in Fort Lauderdale, Fla.

Dr. Konin has worked in numerous high school, college, clinic, and professional environments. His experiences have included providing care at NASCAR and rodeo events, the Olympic training center in Lake Placid, NY, professional baseball spring training, the American Basketball Association (ABA), professional baseball summer camps, and serving on the track and field medical staff for the 1996 Atlanta Committee for the Olympic Games.

Dr. Konin is and has been very involved in the athletic training profession. He has served as the Vice President and Newsletter Editor for the Delaware Athletic Trainers' Association, and as a member of the Examining Board for Physical Therapy in the state of Delaware. He has also been a committee member for the National Athletic Trainers' Association's (NATA) Clinical/Industrial/Corporate athletic trainer's committee and the reimbursement advisory group. For a number of years, Jeff was the NATA's liason to the American Physical Therapy Association.

Dr. Konin has published numerous articles on various topics in the areas of sports medicine, athletic training, and physical therapy. He resides in Harrisonburg, Va with his wife Gina and two sons, KJ and Christopher.

Margaret A. Frederick, MS, ATC, is the Coordinator of Clinical Education and an Instructor in the Athletic Training Education Program at Longwood University in Farmville, Virginia. She holds a BS degree in Health Science with a concentration in Athletic Training from James Madison University, where she also earned a Master's of Science degree in Kinesiology. Ms. Frederick is currently pursuing a Doctorate of Education degree from the University of South Carolina.

A certified athletic trainer for more than a dozen years, she has experience as a high school athletic trainer and as an educator at the undergraduate and master's levels. Other professional roles include serving as secretary of the Virginia Athletic Trainers' Association and test site administrator for the NATABOC certification examination. Ms. Frederick lives in Richmond, Va.

Contributing Authors

Todd Babcock, MS, ATC
The SPORT CLINIC
Riverside, California

Nikki Beil, ATC
Richmond, Virginia

Dan Campbell, PT/ATR
Coordinator of Athletic Training Services
Mayo Clinic Sports Medicine
Rochester, Minnesota

Tamerah N. Hunt, MS, ATC, CSCS
Graduate Assistant Athletic Trainer
The University of Georgia
Athens, Georgia

John Kaltenborn, MS, ATC
Assistant Athletic Trainer, Instructor
James Madison University
Harrisonburg, Virginia

Karen M. Lew, MEd., ATC, LAT
Program Director
Athletic Training Education
Southeastern Louisiana University
Hammond, Louisianna

Sheila K. Nicholson, Esq., MBA, PT
Associate at Quintairos, Prieto, Wood & Boyer, P.A. Law Firm
Tampa, Florida

PREFACE

The profession of athletic training has led the way amongst health care providers for many years, serving a role as the first responder. Over time, the first responder role evolved into the daily rehabilitation specialist, the confidant, and much more. Of all of the responsibilities of today's certified athletic trainer, most overlooked has been the need for adequate, proper, legal, and timely documentation.

The increase in the number of physically active individuals being treated by certified athletic trainers is merely one reason for the challenges associated with daily documentation. The lack of thorough and formal training through previous historical methods of classroom instruction has also left today's certified athletic trainer without necessary skills in some employment settings. The rapid advancement of access to electronic information has also posed challenges to today's practicing certified athletic trainer. Perhaps the single greatest impetus for advancing one's documentation skill set lies in the overwhelming fear of litigation that potentially shadows each and every clinical incidence.

Regardless of fear and change, the need to document appropriately is a fundamental survival skill for the health care provider. Documentation is THE method of written communication amongst and between certified athletic trainers, athletic training students, allied health care providers, physicians, administrators, parents, and others. With this broad spectrum of people in the information loop, the need for a variety of documentation forms is substantiated.

For many years now, the athletic training profession has taken the luxury of borrowing documentation designed for other allied health professions. In recent years, textbooks written for athletic trainers on topics ranging from organization and administration to rehabilitation have included brief sections on methods of documentation. To date, however, none have specifically been written in stand-alone form with the certified athletic trainer in mind. To our knowledge, this book becomes the first to do so.

The primary intent of this book is to meet the needs of today's athletic training student across the curriculum. It is clearly recognized that few, if any, athletic training education programs will have a stand-alone course that teaches the principles of documentation. Rather, various components of proper documentation are introduced and implemented throughout one's academic sequence of courses. In fact, the building of documentation knowledge as a skill set for the athletic training student serves as an excellent example for how learning over time is embedded in one's experiences.

This workbook is broken down into three main components. First, the seven chapters didactically explain basic principles and styles associated with documentation in athletic training. This information includes the dos and don'ts of medical documentation. The second component provides opportunity for athletic training students to practice their documentation skills. This is presented in the form of discussion questions and worksheets dispersed throughout the book. Finally, an exhaustive appendix provides examples of currently used forms of various kinds in the athletic training setting today. We recognize that most certified athletic trainers are capable of creating their own forms to meet the needs of their workplace. The intent of these examples is to expose athletic training students to the myriad forms of documentation that exist. This will be helpful because many athletic training students gain the majority of their educational experience at their own academic institution, with short stints at affiliated clinical sites, which limits their exposure to different documentation forms.

This text also makes an effort to provide the reader with very practical information. Each chapter contains "pearls of wisdom" specifically designed to serve as condensed synopses of important information. In addition, the "common mistakes" with "suggestions for avoidance" serve to assist the reader throughout the learning curve associated with documentation. Having the wisdom of the mistakes many of us made in our early days of documenting will only lead to a quicker grasp of the written medical language.

As the age of information fiber optically passes by us, there will no doubt be a need to update the information presented in this text so that the profession of athletic training can do its best to stay in the race for good written communication. As the editors of this text, we do not feel compelled to label ourselves as the experts of documentation. Instead, our intuitive thinking is more related to that of facilitators. As such, we urge the athletic training community, educators and clinicians alike, to enhance their written communication skills and serve as leaders to our athletic training students—the future professionals in our field.

Jeff G. Konin, PhD, ATC, PT
Margaret A. Frederick, MS, ATC

Chapter 1

INTRODUCTION TO DOCUMENTATION

LEARNING OBJECTIVES

Following the completion of this chapter, the reader will be able to:

1. Identify and explain the purposes of medical documentation.
2. Explain the Nagi and International Classification of Impairments, Disabilities, and Handicaps models of disablement and how these conceptual frameworks apply to medical documentation.
3. Explain the effects of applying disablement models to athletic training.

INTRODUCTION

Over the last several decades, health care in the United States has undergone considerable change. Research on new and better treatments for illness and disease has contributed greatly to skyrocketing health care costs. In an effort to control costs, insurance companies have developed strict regulations regarding reimbursement for health care. This has created an environment of harsh competition for the health care dollar. Simultaneously, the liability of health care professionals appears to have increased dramatically. An abundance of lawsuits alleging medical malpractice are filed each year, making the health care professional increasingly vulnerable. Given these trends, the need for effective medical documentation has never been greater.

Athletic trainers have long accepted the necessity and importance of documentation. Standard No. 3 of the National Athletic Trainers' Association Board of Certification Inc. (NATABOC) *Standards of Professional Practice* delineates the responsibility of the athletic trainer in maintaining proper documentation.[1] However, given that athletic trainers are relative newcomers to the battle for third-party reimbursement and that athletic trainers are increasingly vulnerable to lawsuits, there must be a renewed dedication to proficiency in medical documentation and to the implementation of effective medical documentation systems.

PURPOSE OF MEDICAL DOCUMENTATION

Generally speaking, medical documentation can be defined as any data that is recorded in a patient's medical record. Medical documentation serves as the official record of the care provided to the patient.[2,3] Evaluation forms, medical referrals, progress notes, test results, and health history forms are but a few examples of medical documentation. Common types of medical documentation utilized by athletic trainers include pre-participation physical exam forms, initial evaluations, daily progress notes, physician's notes, informed consent, and rehabilitation logs. A medical documentation system refers to the organization and administration of the policies and processes related to medical documentation. The athletic trainer must be proficient in both medical documentation and in organizing and administrating the medical documentation system.

The ultimate goal of the athletic trainer is the provision of high-quality health care for athletes and the physically active. Documentation helps ensure quality health care in a number of ways.

> In order for medical documentation to be effective, a medical documentation system must be developed based on (1) the mission of the facility, (2) a conceptual framework, and (3) the needs of patient/athletes.

Communication

The athletic trainer's most valuable asset is the ability to communicate. Effective documentation facilitates the athletic trainer's communication with other members of the sports medicine team, such as physicians, physical therapists, nurses, parents, and coaches.

Organization

Documentation helps the athletic trainer organize the patient/athlete's medical data. For example, information gathered during an initial injury evaluation must be recorded so that another health care professional can read the evaluation and determine exactly what data was collected. By facilitating communication, well-organized medical documentation can positively impact the quality of patient/athlete care. Also, documentation aids the athletic trainer in clinical decision making. In completing appropriate documentation, the athletic trainer is required to organize not only the data but also the thought processes related to patient/athlete care.[4] Organized documentation helps the athletic trainer make better decisions.

Quality Assurance

There is an old adage that, "Experience is the best teacher." That statement could be reworded to read, "The more experience you have, the better athletic trainer you are." Yet, practically speaking, experience alone is not a valid measure of athletic training proficiency. The athletic trainer should periodically review and analyze documentation of patient/athlete cases to glean objective information about the effectiveness of specific treatments. Ergo, athletic trainers must avoid the philosophy, "That's the way I've always treated that injury," and focus instead on the objective evidence that a treatment is effective for an illness or injury. Effectiveness is determined by reviewing the medical documentation of a patient/athlete's subjective and objective responses to a treatment or treatment plan.

The medical documentation system should include a process for reviewing records. Peer review of medical records can help ensure high standards of quality in both medical documentation and patient/athlete care. While the high standard of care will improve the outcome for the patient/athlete, quality medical documentation will ensure a higher rate of third-party payment and also provide a better defense in case of legal action against the athletic trainer. Third-party payers (insurance companies) generally conduct another type of medical record review. The purpose of this review is usually to determine if the insurance will reimburse the provider for patient/athlete care. Although third-party payment for athletic training services is still more the exception than the rule, a growing number of athletic trainers are already billing for services and that trend is expected to continue.

Outcomes Research

As previously stated, medical documentation provides objective evidence of the efficacy of a treatment or treatment plan. Advancement of the athletic training profession depends largely on the ability to prove that athletic training services are effective (eg, have positive outcomes). Effective documentation of the patient/athlete's subjective and objective responses to a treatment or treatment plan enhances the validity and reliability of the evidence (data). Researchers can then use the data to establish relationships between treatments and outcomes, which will further inform the practice of athletic training.

Reimbursement

Effective documentation is essential to obtaining third-party reimbursement for athletic training services. Standards and guidelines for documentation are established by third-party payers and are generally based on regulations set by the Centers for Medicare and Medicaid Services (CMS), formerly known as the Health Care Financing Administration (HCFA).[5] The athletic trainer must adhere to the appropriate standards and guidelines to ensure a high rate of reimbursement. This topic is covered in depth in Chapter 6.

> In high school and collegiate athletic training settings, a calendar is a very useful tool to assist with collecting and maintaining documentation. Mark a calendar with due dates for paperwork such as pre-participation examination forms, post-season health history questionnaires, etc. There are likely to be several different due dates, based on the various sports' competitive seasons.

Liability

The athletic trainer should always bear in mind that effective medical documentation is the first line of defense in a lawsuit. In many cases, medical documentation is the main source of objective evidence of patient/athlete care.[6] Medical records are permanent, legal documents. Thus, the athletic trainer must avoid recording false, exaggerated, or fabricated data. It would be prudent to assume that a lawyer will scrutinize every patient/athlete file and each document therein. As a health care professional, the athletic trainer should adopt a common health care mantra, "not documented, not done." Legal aspects of documentation are discussed in detail in Chapter 5.

Athletic Training Services Usage Patterns

Another purpose of documentation is to track the number and types of athletic training services provided in a specific time period.[7] This data can be useful in a variety of ways, including determining injury incidence patterns, cost/benefit analysis, and budget needs. Tracking the volume of patient cases and billing associated with athletic training services can assist in making personnel decisions.

Marketing Tool

The role of marketing and public relations in the practice of athletic training is often overlooked and ignored. Yet, a proactive and focused marketing plan can greatly enhance the practice of athletic training. First, medical documentation can be used to track referral sources. Identifying patterns of referral can help inform the marketing plan. Secondly, effective documentation can be used to enhance patient/athlete communication, leading to increased customer satisfaction.[2] Satisfied customers are an invaluable marketing resource.

Legislative Requirements

Athletic trainers may be required by state law to maintain documentation. Athletic trainers should consult the state agency that administrates the law in the state where he or she practices to determine documentation requirements.

To summarize, effective medical documentation is valuable for a variety of reasons. The athletic trainer must be proficient in documentation skills in order to communicate effectively, help reduce the risk of liability, and uphold the standards and guidelines of the NATABOC, state practice acts, and third-party payers. The athletic trainer must also be able to organize and administer a medical documentation system.

CONCEPTUAL FRAMEWORK FOR DOCUMENTATION

In order for documentation to be effective, a conceptual framework must be developed, and the documentation policy and procedures must be embedded in that framework. The key role of any conceptual framework is to identify the concepts and relationships in a complex phenomenon. Creating the conceptual framework establishes a common language in order to clarify meaning and enhance communication about a particular entity. Many conceptual frameworks have been developed to create a common language for describing health status and disability. Three of the most commonly-used health and disability models are presented in this chapter.

The Nagi Model of Disablement, developed by noted sociologist Saad Nagi in the 1960s, contains 4 key concepts: active pathology, physical impairment, functional limitation and disability.[8,9,10] A description of the Nagi Model is presented in Table 1-1.

In 1980, the World Health Organization (WHO) developed the ICIDH in order to create a common language for describing and understanding health and health status.[10,11] This framework has 4 basic components: disease, impairment, disability, and handicap. Table 1-2 contains a description of the ICIDH model.

Table 1-1	Nagi Model of Disablement			
	Active Pathology	*Impairment*	*Functional Limitation*	*Disability*
Definition	The intrinsic pathology or disorder	Anatomical, physiological, mental, or emotional abnormality or loss	Limitation of performance at the level of the whole organism or person	Limitation in performance of socially defined roles and tasks within a sociocultural and physical environment
Frame of Reference	Cell	Tissue, organ, body system	Whole person	External environment/ culture/ society
Example: Point guard on basketball team sustains 3 degree ACL tear	3 degree ACL tear	+ Lachman's test Knee Flexion 80 degrees	Inability to run Inability to jump	Unable to play basketball

Based on Jette AM. Physical disablement concepts for physical therapy research and practice. *Phys Ther*. 1994;74(5):11-18.

The ICIDH model has been continually revised since its inception. The most recent version of the ICIDH is the International Statistical Classification of Diseases and Related Health Problems Version 10 (ICD-10), adopted by WHO in 1999.[11] This biomedical model is used to classify a person's level of disease or disability, and does not account for social, psychological, or cultural aspects of disease. In 2001, WHO adopted the International Classification of Functioning, Disability and Health (ICF), to be used in collaboration with ICD-10.[1] ICF is a comprehensive framework for describing health status and disability that integrates biomedical and psychosocial theories of disease. ICD-10 is mainly intended to classify diagnoses and diseases, while ICF is more focused on health status and the factors that influence health status. WHO notes that "ICD-10 and ICF are therefore complementary, and users are encouraged to utilize these 2 members of the WHO family of international classifications together."[11]

Similarities between ICF and Nagi are obvious. "Active pathology" is synonymous with "health condition." "Impairments" are similar to "body functions and structure." "Activity" is essentially the same thing as "functional limitation," just as participation is the same as "disability." However, the ICF model emphasizes the influence of "contextual factors," which are not incorporated in the Nagi model. Examples of contextual factors include the physical environment in which a person lives (eg, urban vs. rural) and psychological aspects of disease (depression vs. positive mental attitude). Figure 1-1 illustrates the ICF model.

When documentation policy and process are embedded in a framework such as Nagi or ICF, both the athletic trainer and the patient/athlete will benefit. Perhaps the most important application of a disablement model is to help structure the evaluation, treatment, and rehabilitation of musculoskeletal injuries. Most athletic trainers spend a majority of their time carrying out these functions. Focusing on a patient/athlete's disability, rather than simply a set of signs and symptoms or test results, is similar to seeing the forest instead of the trees. That is, the athletic trainer must recognize that the goal of a particular treatment plan is to address and correct a patient/athlete's inability to participate in a particular activity, not strictly to restore range of motion to a joint or strength to a muscle. This shift in thinking should result in a better outcome for the patient/athlete, since the treatment plan will, at its core, be tailored to the individual, not to the injury. Application of a disablement model to the documentation of the evaluation, treatment, and rehabilitation of musculoskeletal injuries will have the added benefit of providing the athletic trainer with feedback about the success of particular treatment and rehabilitation protocols. The athlet-

Table 1-2	International Classification of Impairments, Disabilities, and Handicaps Model			
	Disease	*Impairment*	*Disability*	*Handicap*
Definition	Biochemical, physiologic, and anatomical abnormalities of the human organism	Loss or abnormality at the tissue, organ, or body system level	Inability to perform a task or participate in activity considered normal for a human being	Disadvantage for a given individual, resulting from an impairment or a disability that limits or prevents the fulfillment of a role that is normal (depending on age, sex, and ocial and cultural factors) for that individual
Frame of reference	Cell	Tissue, organ, body system	Whole person, external environment, culture	Society (not the individual)
Example: Point guard on basketball team sustains 3 degree ACL tear	3 degree ACL tear	+ Lachman's test Knee Flexion 80 degrees	Inability to run Inability to jump	Inability to play basketball

Based on Jette AM. Physical disablement concepts for physical therapy research and practice. *Phys Ther*. 1994;74(5):11-18.

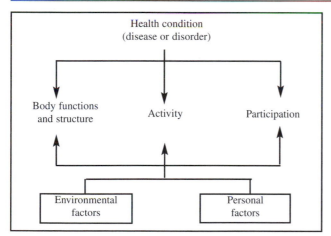

Figure 1-1. International Classification of Functioning, Disability and Health (ICF) model developed by WHO to describe health status. (World Health Organization. Towards a common language for functioning, disability and health: ICF. Geneva, 2002. Available at: http://www3.who.int/icf/icftemplate.cfm. Accessed on January 26, 2004.)

ic trainer will benefit from this structure and from the feedback that is inherent in this type of documentation.

In summary, medical documentation is more important today than ever before in health care. Documentation serves a multitude of purposes, including communication, organization, patient/athlete management, quality assurance, reimbursement, outcomes research, marketing, and usage patterns. A conceptual framework is necessary to define and clarify the policy and process of documentation. The Nagi Model of Disablement and the two WHO models are among the most commonly used frameworks for describing health status. Application of one of the models will greatly enhance the quality of athletic training services, when used appropriately by athletic trainers.

REFERENCES

1. NATABOC Standards of Professional Practice. Available at: http://www.bocatc.org. Accessed January 25, 2004.
2. Baeten AM, Moran ML, Phillipi LM. *Documenting Physical Therapy: The Reviewer Perspective*. Woburn, Mass: Butterworth-Heinemann; 1999.

Common Mistake #1

Not tracking athletic training room usage patterns

Suggestion for avoidance: Use a treatment log sheet, electronic spreadsheet, or database to track numbers and types of treatments provided in the athletic training room. This will help justify budget, personnel decisions, and capital improvements.

Common Mistake #2

Not conducting review and analysis of athletic training services, especially outcomes assesment and medical records review

Suggestion for avoidance: The administrator of the facility should be responsible for overseeing annual review and analysis of athletic training services. This role is essential to maintaining high quality athletic health care services.

Common Mistake #3

Disorganized medical documentation in the athletic training facility

Suggestion for avoidance: Using standardized forms can help the athletic trainer organize notes taken during evaluations and treatments. Commerical injury tracking software can be used to organize all aspects of documentation, including health history questionnaires, preparticipation exam results, injury records, and treatment records.

3. Lukan M. *Documentation for Physical Therapy Assistants*. 2nd ed. Philadelphia: FA Davis; 2001.

4. Kettenbach G. *Writing SOAP Notes: With Patient/Client Management Formats*. 3rd ed. Philadelphia: FA Davis; 2004.

5. Centers for Medicare and Medicaid Services. Medicare Learning Network (Medlearn): Documentation Guidelines —Evaluation and Management Services. Available at: http://www.cms.hhs.gov/medlearn/emdoc.asp. Accessed January 25, 2004.

6. Scott RW. *Legal Aspects of Documenting Patient Care*. Gaithersburg, Md: Aspen Publishers Inc.; 1994.

7. Rankin JM, Ingersoll, CD. *Athletic Training Management: Concepts and Applications*. 2nd ed. Champaign, Ill: Human Kinetics Publishers; 2001.

8. Nagi SZ. *Disability and Rehabilitation: Legal, Clinical and Self-concepts and Measurement*. Ohio State University Press; 1969: 10-17.

9. Nagi SZ. Disability in America: toward a national agenda for prevention. In: Pope AM, Tarlov AR, eds. *Disability in America: Toward A National Agenda for Prevention*. Washington, DC: National Academy Press; 1991.

10. Jette AM. Physical disablement concepts for physical therapy research and practice. *Phys Ther*. 1994;74(5):11-18.

11. World Health Organization. Towards a common language for functioning, disability and health: ICF. Geneva, 2002. Available at: http://www3.who.int/icf/icftemplate.cfm. Accessed January 26, 2004.

DISCUSSION ITEMS

Using the information presented in this chapter, answer the following:

1. What do you feel is the most important reason for efficient and thorough documentation in the athletic training environment?

2. Do you think there is a difference in the way athletic trainers document based upon setting? What differences might exist between high school, clinical, and university settings?

3. In your academic setting, what are some examples of how you have witnessed athletic trainers documenting various aspects of medical care?

Konin JG, Frederick MA. *Documentation for Athletic Training*. Thorofare, NJ: SLACK Incorporated; 2005.

Chapter 2

Basic Principles
of Medical Documentation

Learning Objectives

Following the completion of this chapter, the reader will be able to:

1. Identify and explain the principles of medical documentation.
2. Describe the documentation standard set forth in the National Athletic Trainers Association Board of Certification *Standards of Professional Practice*.
3. Describe how to record physician's verbal orders in a medical record.

Introduction

Standards and guidelines for medical documentation have been established by a variety of organizations, including the Centers for Medicare and Medicaid Services (CMS).[1] The largest third-party payer in the United States, CMS sets standards and guidelines for medical documentation for participating health care providers, such as physicians and hospitals.[1] Health care professions, such as nursing and physical therapy, also establish standards and guidelines for documentation. The significance of the CMS requirements is that they are regarded as the gold standard and are often adapted for use by other third-party payers (insurance companies). So if the athletic trainer seeks reimbursement for services, the CMS standards and guidelines, or similar rules, may apply.

In the NATABOC Standards of Professional Practice, documentation is addressed.[2] Standard No. 3 reads as follows:

The athletic trainer shall accept responsibility for recording details of the athlete's health status. Documentation shall include:

1. Athlete's name and any other identifying information
2. Referral source (doctor, dentist)
3. Date, initial assessment, results, and database
4. Program plan and estimated length
5. Program methods, results, and revisions
6. Date of discontinuation and summary
7. Athletic trainer's signature

Since documents such the NATABOC *Standards of Professional Practice* are used to establish the standard of care for athletic trainers, the athletic trainer is obligated to adhere to the guidelines above. Further discussion of NATA documentation guidelines and professional standards are presented in the appendix section.

While documentation standards and guidelines vary among health care settings, certain principles are commonly held as essential to all types of medical documentation because the medical record is a legal document. These rules are derived from the various documentation standards and guidelines in health care, as well as legal, statutes.

Practice, practice, practice. Proficiency in medical documentation requires continual critiquing and refining.

MEDICAL TERMINOLOGY

All health care providers should use appropriate medical terminology in medical documentation.[3] This will enhance communication among all types of health care providers. Types of medical terminology with which the athletic trainer, and all health care professionals, must be familiar include pathology, biomechanics, orthopedics, and musculoskeletal system. For example, body parts should be described using anatomical nomenclature (eg, "tibia" instead of "lower leg"). Movement should be described using correct biomechanical terms (eg, "gait" instead of "walk").

Medical Abbreviations

Medical documentation typically contains myriad abbreviations that, while enhancing efficiency, can contribute to confusion and errors.[4] Many health professions have a list of acceptable abbreviations in an effort to ensure common understanding and alleviate confusion and mistakes. However, this does not fully eliminate the possibility of misunderstanding. Also, time spent learning to use and interpret abbreviations can decrease the efficiency that is often attributed to their use. Patient/athlete safety is of utmost importance and care must be taken that the use of abbreviations in medical records does not compromise this. Another issue with medical abbreviations arises when insurance companies review medical records. The reviewer may not be familiar with the abbreviations, and also may not bother to research the meaning. This can be cause for denial of a claim, which can delay or restrict patient/athlete care and reimbursement for services.[4]

Despite the drawbacks, medical abbreviations are still commonly used. Thus, the athletic trainer should become proficient in using and interpreting medical abbreviations. Health care facilities and insurance companies commonly have specific sets of medical abbreviations. It is incumbent on the athletic trainer to know and understand the medical abbreviations used in his/her practice setting. When there is doubt about comprehension, abbreviations should be avoided.[3,4] Sometimes taking the time to write the whole word will be more efficient in the long term.

Punctuation

Correct punctuation is important to ensure correct interpretation of data in medical records. When writing in narrative style, the athletic trainer should take care to use appropriate sentence structure, including the use of punctuation marks. In other medical documentation such as SOAP notes (which will be discussed in Chapter 4), it is essential that a common usage for various punctuation marks be clearly understood by all interested parties. To ensure common understanding, many facilities include a list of punctuation and how to interpret punctuation along with the list of medical abbreviations.

Avoid using hyphens on evaluation, treatment, and rehabilitation forms. Since the hyphen (-) looks exactly like the negative sign (-), the reader may misunderstand the meaning of the symbol.

Accuracy

Data entered in medical records must never be falsified, exaggerated, or fabricated.[3] The athletic trainer should exercise extreme care in recording data precisely and objectively. Objective measurements and findings are the hallmark of accuracy. One should not necessarily render judgment or opinion unless as done in the assessment component of documented records. The reliability and validity of testing will contribute to accurate documentation. Updating medical records regularly and auditing records will help one improve upon accurate methods of documenting future medical charts. Keeping up with industry standards and legislative and regulatory laws that are passed will also contribute to accuracy with documentation.

Use quotation marks when recording statements made by the patient/athlete, as when taking a medical history.

Brevity

Medical documentation should contain concise, short statements. Phrases joined by the word "and" should also be avoided.[3] Abbreviations can facilitate brevity. However, accuracy and clarity must not be sacrificed for the sake of brevity. The athletic trainer must include all necessary information in a manner that will ensure complete understanding.

Clarity

In order to be effective, a medical document must convey meaning readily. Avoid vague terms, changes in verb tense, and abbreviations that may inhibit comprehension.[3] Document in a medical chart with the anticipation that the next person who reads the chart will need to continue with a previous intervention or follow up with your suggested documented notes. If such terms are not clear or legible, the lack of clarity may ultimately affect the outcome of care provided.

> Avoid leaving empty spaces or lines in medical documentation. This will help reduce the risk of falsifying documents after the fact.

Date and Signature

Every entry in a patient/athlete's medical record should be signed and dated. In the case of a document completed by an athletic training student, the record should be signed by the student and by the supervising ATC. An athletic training student in an accredited curriculum should sign his/her name following the completion of a medical entry as "John Doe, ATS."

Timeliness

The athletic trainer should record data as soon as possible after it has been collected in order to ensure accuracy. This is often a challenge for athletic trainers, given that a number of patient/athletes are typically seen in a short period of time. In order to facilitate the timely recording of data, the athletic trainer should always keep a pen and small notepad handy. Shorthand notes jotted down quickly during or after an evaluation or treatment can help ensure accuracy when completing the documentation at a later time. It is absolutely essential, however, that the ath-

> Record only what you observe and what the patient/athlete tells you. Avoid embellishing or inferring meaning.

letic trainer make time to completely and accurately record all evaluations, treatments, and rehab sessions. Jotting down shorthand notes should not be a substitute for appropriate documentation.

Language

When writing medical documentation, the athletic trainer should use professional language. This includes the use of medical terminology and accepted abbreviations where appropriate. Personal pronouns (I, we, you, he, she) should not be used in medical documentation. Medical documentation should be focused on the patient/athlete, not the athletic trainer. Personal opinion is highly inappropriate in medical documentation.

> Sign every entry you make in a patient/athlete's medical record.

RECORDING VERBAL PHYSICIAN ORDERS

Athletic trainers practice under the supervision of physicians, and, therefore, communicate with physicians regularly. This relationship is mutually beneficial to all parties, including the patient/athlete. One result of this relationship is that physicians will give verbal orders, either in person or via the telephone, to the athletic trainer in regard to a specific patient/athlete. It is incumbent on the athletic trainer to record these orders, as issued, in the patient/athlete's medical record. When recording verbal orders, the exact order, time, and date should be included. The athletic trainer should indicate the name of the physician, and should then sign the order. The physician should co-sign verbal orders as soon as possible after the order is issued, perhaps during on-campus rounds or during a routine meeting with the athletic trainer.[3]

Correcting Mistakes

Data must never be erased or eliminated from a medical record using correction fluid or other method. The athletic trainer should correct mistakes by drawing a single line through the error and then initializing the correction. It is a good idea to get in the habit of also noting the date of the correction:

pulsed JGK 1/31/04

Rx consisted of US 1.2w/cm^2 ~~cont~~ for 5' to the Lt patella tendon.

Common Mistake #1

Recording what you think the patient/athlete is trying to say instead of recording exactly what was said

Suggestion for avoidance: Use verbatim quotes when appropriate. Remember that making inferences about meaning constitutes falsification of the medical document.

Common Mistake #2

Using vague terms such as "moderate swelling" and "significant pain"

Suggestion for avoidance: Prefabricated forms can help the athletic trainer remember to use objective measures when recording information. Use documentation forms that include pain scales or questionnaires. Use documentation forms that prompt the measurement of edema and effusion.

Common Mistake #3

Using so many abbreviations that the note is unclear and confusing

Suggestion for avoidance: Use only those abbreviations that are approved by the facility and/or by the third-party payer. A list of acceptable abbreviations should be provided to all health care professionals in the facility, in order to facilitate communication and avoid misunderstanding. If an abbreviation may be misunderstood, always write out the entire word. Review records written by peers, and have peers review your records, to screen for confusing phrases and abbreviations.

When the above mentioned guidelines are followed, the result should be accurate, clear, concise medical documentation recorded the same way for every patient/athlete. Standardization is key in maintaining high quality medical documentation. The athletic trainer should develop proficiency in medical documentation such that each entry in each medical record is recorded with the same quality. This will help ensure that each patient/athlete enjoys the benefits of appropriate medical documentation discussed in this chapter.

REFERENCES

1. Centers for Medicare and Medicaid Services. Medicare Learning Network (Medlearn): Documentation Guidelines—Evaluation and Management Services. Available at: http://www.cms.hhs.gov/medlearn/emdoc.asp. Accessed January 25, 2004.

2. NATABOC Standards of Professional Practice. Available at: www.nataboc.org. Accessed January 25, 2004.

3. Kettenbach G. *Writing SOAP notes: With Patient/Client Management Formats.* 3rd ed. Philadelphia: FA Davis; 2004.

4. Lukan M. *Documentation for Physical Therapy Assistants.* 2nd ed. Philadelphia: FA Davis; 2001.

DISCUSSION ITEMS

Using the information presented in this chapter, answer the following:

1. How would you write a medical note of any kind that would be inclusive of the standards endorsed by the NATABOC?

2. Can you think of some medical abbreviations that you have seen used in the athletic training setting that have multiple meanings?

3. Do you have any suggestions for creating a medical abbreviation for a word or term commonly used in the athletic training profession that would not be confusing to others in its abbreviated version?

4. What mistakes have you witnessed with documentation in your own university or college setting?

5. Look through Appendix B. What words or terms do you find to be confusing? What words or terms do you see used differently in your clinical experiences?

Konin JG, Frederick MA. *Documentation for Athletic Training.* Thorofare, NJ: SLACK Incorporated; 2005.

Chapter 3

TYPES OF WRITTEN DOCUMENTATION

LEARNING OBJECTIVES

Following the completion of this chapter, the reader will be able to:

1. Differentiate between a variety of written documentation and their uses.
2. Understand the need for written documentation.
3. Observe several examples of written documentation and templates for future use in an athletic training facility.

INTRODUCTION

The ever-evolving medical field requires us to document for a variety of reasons. These may include, but are certainly not limited to, accuracy of treatments, legal issues, continuity of care, outcomes results, and procedural concerns of the facility where the treatment is being performed. The purpose of this chapter is to introduce and explain some of the many examples of written forms of documentation that an athletic trainer may come across in clinical, educational, and administrative practice.

INITIAL EVALUATION FORMS

The initial evaluation is the key to the introduction of the patient and will assist in developing an accurate assessment of an injury or illness. The evaluation process also formulates a list of patient problems and goals that can then be established and directed toward an appropriate and timely treatment intervention.

The more immediate the evaluation occurs, the easier it is to assess the situation and chief complaint of the patient/athlete. The initial evaluation should include a systematic approach so details may be better accrued and not omitted. An example of an initial evaluation form for the

October 20, 2004

Dear Dr. Smith,

We have treated John Gooden for approximately 3 weeks following an acute episode of lateral epicondylitis to his right elbow at the beginning of his tennis season.
Treatment has consisted of active and passive stretching, ultrasound, muscular strengthening, and a gradual progression of activity.
His pain has subsided from a 6/10 to a 3/10 during this time, and his strength with elbow and wrist extension on the involved side has both increased to 4/5. He has minimal palpable tenderness and no observable swelling. There are no range of motion limitations.
It appears as though we have met our goals of decreasing his pain and improving upon his strength in the elbow. He has also been able to return to participation, hitting 25 serves, 20 forehands, and 15 backhands daily pain-free.
Thank you for your assistance in evaluating Mr. Gooden. We will inform you of any further progression or change in his status.

Sincerely,

Jeff G. Konin (signed)

Jeff G. Konin, PhD, ATC, PT

Figure 3-1. Example of a progress note.

knee is in Appendix H. Subjective information from the patient/athlete, as well as others, is as critical as the information that you are able to assess as part of the evaluation. All of these pieces of information need to be identified as part of an initial evaluation document.

The writing of the initial evaluation is the critical aspect. You must remember to include everything and anything that is relevant to the injury and provide only factual information; the information should be clearly written and easily read by other health care practitioners. Once the evaluation is complete and a plan of treatment is implemented, it is important for the athletic trainer to maintain and update progress notes throughout the entire treatment until the injury has healed or the patient has been discharged.

Progress Notes

Progress notes are a form of documentation used to update all interested parties in the status of a patient/athlete. Progress notes can be used to record the changes that an individual is making. The progress note can be drafted in many styles. It should include the current status of the person, current treatment interventions applied, objective measurements and subjective reports of the patient, as well as long-term and short-term goals that are both temporal and measurable. It is important to both quantify and qualify the goals being stated in the progress notes (Figure 3-1).

Discharge Notes

A discharge note is a final version of a progress note that identifies a written termination of treatment interven-

tions for an individual. As a person is ready to reenter activity or be released from treatment, a discharge note is helpful in ensuring complete understanding by all parties of the status of a patient/athlete's condition. A discharge note should contain current ability as well as measurements. A final statement regarding the prognosis should be included (Figure 3-2).

Discharge notes are recorded by an athletic trainer when a patient has reached long-term goals and will no longer be receiving treatment on a regular basis for a specific injury or illness. These notes are intended to contain the patient's condition at the time of discharge as well as a summary of the rehabilitation protocol and its duration. Included in the discharge note should be records of the patient's response to specific treatments and their compliance. A copy of the discharge note should be kept in the patient's medical file for future reference.

Flow Chart

Flow charts are often used within a patient's chart as a quick and efficient means to record treatment interventions without duplicating written statements. Rather than writing and rewriting similar notes, a flow chart allows for a quick glance at successive interventions in a graph-like format. This format often lists the date and the exercise or treatment intervention along the "x" and "y" axis, and the corresponding connecting box represents the parameters of the intervention (Figure 3-3).

All personal opinions need to be omitted from objective medical records. If you are unsure, leave it out.

October 20, 2004

Dear Dr. Smith,

Sarah Barnes has been seen in our sports medicine department daily for the past 6 weeks following her left knee partial medial menisectomy.
Sarah has progressed nicely, to date presenting with full pain-free active and passive range of motion. Knee flexion and extension are 95% compared bilaterally with isokinetic testing at all speeds and parameters. There is no joint effusion.
Sarah is now able to return to golf with no restrictions. As a result, we plan to discharge her from our formal care so that she can return to playing golf full-time.
If you have any questions please contact me. Thank you for your assistance in her care.

Sincerely,

Jeff G. Konin (signed)

Jeff G. Konin, PhD, ATC, PT

Figure 3-2. Example of a discharge note.

Athlete's Name _____   Sport _____
Injury _____   L   R

Exercise	Knee Ext	Leg Curl	Squat	Hip Abd SLR	Hip Abd SLR	Quad sets	Toe Raise	Ham Stretch	Cyro
Date									
10/15/04	3x10 15#	2x10 10#	4x10	3x10 3#	3x10 4#	25	10xbw	5x	15'
10/16/04	4x10 15#	2x10 10#	5x10	3x10 3#	4x10 4#	25	10xbw	5x	15'
10/17/04	4x10	3x10	3x10	4x10	5x10	30	15xbw	5x	20'

Figure 3-3. Example of a flow chart.

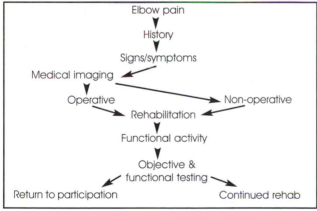

Figure 3-4. Example of an algorithm chart.

Algorithm Chart

An algorithm chart is a series of "if-then" statements that are used to determine treatment procedures or actions. This type of chart can be helpful for beginning athletic trainers or new employees to follow as they are designing a rehabilitation protocol or dealing with an emergency situation. Emergency action plans are often created as flow charts. Flow charts are usually easy to follow and have a predetermined set of instructions for the task at hand. They serve to provide a predetermined path for the user to follow, which allows a simple means by which to accomplish a task (Figure 3-4).

Ordinarily flow charts are used to assist with a specific injury or situation. The most common flowcharts used in athletic training facility are for unconscious athletes. They provide the athletic trainer with a step-by-step procedure of what to do and when, by answering either yes or no to the question. A predetermined flow chart will allow athletic trainers to have something to help them follow an appropriate method when providing treatment and making critical decisions.

Always sign and date entries. Being able to retrieve health history information and identifying a sequence of events is a valuable process in decision making.

Physician Letters

Physician letters are becoming more common in athletic training. With new laws and guidelines regarding confidentiality, the athletic trainer, institution, or facility should set up a standard protocol that the physicians are to follow when treating their respective athletes. It may be difficult to obtain physician letters from physicians that are not part of the institution's sports medicine team. If the team physicians are treating an athlete in their own office, it is a good idea to make sure that the athlete's chart identifies him/her as an athlete. The identification can serve as a means for the physician to make certain that a letter is sent to the athletic trainer at the institution. An example of a physician's referral letter is found in Appendix I.

All physicians prefer different formats of letter writing to read. In writing a physician letter, the letter should outline the personal data of the athlete as well as any other information the physician would like to include. Providing basic information such as the injury itself and the initial date of occurrence helps a physician quickly recollect the scenario. The personal data should include the athlete's name, age, injured body part, sport, as well as chief complaint. Most physicians write their letters using the History, Observation, Palpation, Special tests (HOPS) outline and include their findings and instructions for treatment.

In using the HOPS format, it is easy for the athletic trainer to have the specific information needed from the physician. If a letter is sent automatically for every athlete that is treated, it will reduce the amount of time the physician will have to spend on the phone with the athletic trainer. In addition to being more time efficient, it may also help in the accuracy of treatments. The letter should also indicate if and when any return visits are required.

The letter should be kept in the athlete's personal medical folder along with their treatment records and any other pertinent information related to their injury. The athletic trainer can refer to this letter if a need arises. Having documentation of all physician visits insures accuracy in the athlete's records should they be needed in the future.

Injury Report

The injury report can be used for a variety of reasons. It is used to update coaches and the athletic training staff, and as a means for record keeping. An injury report should be updated on a daily basis. The most important information on the injury report should include the athlete's name, the type of injury, the limitations of the injury, and the rehabilitation or treatments the athlete is undergoing. The injury report should be self-explanatory and written

JMU SPORTS MEDICINE		
Daily Injury Report: Softball Date: 10/14/04		

1. *Lisa Younger (ankle sprain)*
2. *Naomi Broadhurst (foot contusion)*
3.

Participation Status

No Practice	Practice Limited
1. *Lisa Younger*	1. *Amy Washburn*
2. *Naomi Broadhurst*	2.
3.	3.

Practice to Tolerance	Remove from injury list
1. *Cindy Hoffman*	1.
2. *Leslie McDougal*	2.

Figure 3-5 Example of injury report.

in terms that all who are intended to read will understand (Figure 3-5).

If someone other than an athletic trainer is reading the injury report, they should be able to see what progress the athlete is making. It should also give the coach or whoever is reading it an indication of whether or not the athlete has been compliant with the treatments. Injury reports, like all other forms of documentation, must remain confidential; athletic trainers should have prior written approval by an patient/athlete to dispense to all parties involved.

Medical History Form

A medical history form is designed to gather information regarding an individual's personal and family medical history. It is important to specify that all previous injuries and illnesses, regardless of when and how they occurred, should be included in the history. In addition to having the patient fill out the history, it is a good idea to discuss it with him or her. Discussing the history with the patient allows him or her to explain anything to you and allows you to take notes and further investigate his or her medical condition (see Appendix E for examples of information forms).

> Always read your documentation for clarity, understanding, and readability. If it is not legible, it does not serve an efficient and effective purpose.

The medical history portion of a preparticipation physical exam should be the most extensive aspect of the exam. Having documentation of previous or current conditions will assist in ensuring the athlete receives appropriate medical care. Questioning for the medical history can be done in a yes/no format but should include space for the athlete to provide explanation. The questions should not be limited to strictly orthopedic questions, but should also include general medical, current medication, psychological treatment, previous surgeries, and anything that may be helpful to the sports medicine team.

Preparticipation Physical Examination

Preparticipation physical exams are a required component for all active athletes. Rules and regulations regarding the preparticipation physical exam are established by the sponsoring organization, and vary greatly. An athlete should be required to have an annual evaluation by a medical doctor, including a thorough assessment and documentation of all body systems. Preparticipation exams are conducted in a variety of ways. All should include similar information accumulation in such a manner that clearly identifies factual status of all body systems; documentation of preexisting injuries and illnesses; and statements relating to whether one is fully cleared, cleared with restrictions, or not cleared to participate. A physician should sign the document clearing the patient/athlete for participation, noting any limitation or deviations from normal that were found during the physical examination (see Appendix E).

CONFIDENTIALITY AGREEMENTS

Confidentiality is important to protect the privacy and dignity of each and every individual (Figure 3-6). The need for confidentiality extends far beyond medical documentation. The athletic trainer is in a position of having knowledge considered to be very personal to a patient. Others may want to know this information for various reasons, and it must be kept confidential and under tight seal. Most facilities require all employees and anyone coming into contact with patients to sign a confidentiality statement that clearly identifies the appropriate and inappropriate use of sharing information. It is necessary to obtain an appropriate release prior to giving out any personal information, whether it be requested by other practitioners, coaches, athletic training students, media, or even family members of those not considered to be minors. If ever in doubt, it is best not to provide information until completely sure of the consent needed.

Medical Release

A medical release and waiver should be signed by all participants regardless of the type of activity they are participating in as an athlete. The release should be reviewed by the institution to insure that it complies with local, state, and federal guidelines. An explanation of risks should be included as well. One of the purposes of this release is to hold the institution and all associated entities harmless for any injury or damages that the athlete may suffer during his or her voluntary participation in athletics (Figure 3-7).

The medical consent form is a legal document signed by the athlete if 18 years of age or older and by a parent or guardian if the athlete is a minor. The statement the athlete is signing allows him or her to receive medical treatment from a physician or any other health care provider that is associated with the athletic program. Any evaluations, treatments, or diagnoses may be given to the parties specified in the release form. Also included in the release is a statement that will allow the athletic trainer to release requested medical information to individuals that may require this information. The athlete has the right to refuse his or her personal and medical information being released to anyone. If the athlete chooses not to grant permission for release of information, he or she should clearly indicate this decision on the medical consent form. The athlete also has the right to change his or her mind at anytime regarding the release of confidential information.

Medical Disqualification

A patient/athlete may be deemed unfit to participate for a multitude of reasons. The health care practitioner must outline the reason for disqualification, providing the athlete with an appropriate form that documents the reason he or she is being disqualified. As an athletic trainer, you must abide by whatever judgement is made by the team physician or physician that issues the disqualification. From the standpoint of documentation, it is always better to have a paper record of why the athlete is being disqualified. Such forms and information provided will be reviewed by appropriate officials who determine disqualification status.

In documenting reasons for disqualification, you must make certain that everything is accurate. The information included in a medical disqualification should include medical exams, diagnostic testing, a written statement from the physician, and any other pertinent materials that would support the disqualifying of an athlete. The disqualification must be based on medical findings and nothing else. Disqualifications must clearly state that an athlete will no longer be able to participate in a given sport.

Fax Cover

As we utilize facsimiles more and more, it is imperative to include a confidentiality statement on the fax cover sheet (Appendix I). Faxing has become a simplistic means to transmit information in a timely manner. If you are fax-

---

Confidentiality Agreement

Confidentiality is a cornerstone of building a strong clinical relationship. As an individual who provides health care you may have access to client's/patient's confidential information that includes biographical data, financial information, medical history and other information. You are expected to protect client confidentiality, privacy and security and to follow these and all associated agency guidelines.

You will use confidential information only as needed to perform duties as a member of the faculty or as a registered student in the athletic training education program. This means, among other things, that:
• You will only access confidential information for which you have a need to know.
• You will respect the confidentiality of any verbal communication or reports printed from any information system containing client's/patient's information and handle, store and dispose of these reports appropriately at the University and associated clinical agency.
• You will not in any way divulge, copy, release, loan, alter, or destroy any confidential information except as properly authorized within the scope of all your professional activities.
• You will carefully protect all confidential information. You will take every precaution so that clients/patients, their families, or other persons do not overhear conversations concerning client/patient care or have the opportunity to view client/patient records.
• You will comply with all policies and procedures and other rules of the University and associated agencies relating to confidentiality of information and access codes.
• You understand that the information accessed through all clinical information systems agencies contains sensitive and confidential client/patient care, business, financial and hospital employee information that should only be disclosed to those authorized to receive it.
• You will not knowingly include or cause to be included in any record or report of false, inaccurate or misleading entry.

You understand that violation of this Confidentiality Agreement may result in disciplinary and legal action with fines. By signing this, you agree that you have read, understand and will comply with the Agreement.

Print Name: _____   Date:_____

Signature: _____   Date: _____

Witness: _____   Date: _____

Figure 3-6. Example of a confidentiality form.

ATHLETIC DEPARTMENT
RELEASE

WHEREBY, I, THE UNDERSIGNED, AM ABOUT TO PARTICIPATE IN A TRY-OUT FOR AN ATHLETIC TEAM UNDER THE SUPERVISION OF THE JEFF'S UNIVERSITY, A STATE OF VIRGINIA INSTITUTION;

WHEREAS, I AM DOING SO ENTIRELY UPON MY OWN INITIATIVE (WITHOUT ANY INCENTIVE OR BEING COERCED), RISK, AND RESPONSIBILITY;

NOW, THEREFORE, IN CONSIDERATION OF THE PERMISSION EXTENDED TO ME TO PARTICIPATE IN THE JEFF'S UNIVERSITY TRY-OUT, I DO HEREBY FOR MYSELF, MY HEIRS, EXECUTORS AND ADMINISTRATORS, REMISE, RELEASE AND FOREVER DISCHARGE AND HOLD HARMLESS JEFF'S UNIVERSITY, ITS COACHES AND ADMINISTRATORS FROM ANY AND ALL CLAIMS, DEMANDS, ACTIONS OR CAUSES OF ACTION ON ACCOUNT OF ANY INJURY TO ME OR ON ACCOUNT OF MY DEATH WHICH MAY OCCUR FROM ANY CAUSE DURING SAID TRY-OUT.

THE ABOVE STATEMENTS APPLY TO THE FOLLOWING:

_____

_____

CANDIDATE SIGNATURE   _____

DATE   _____

_____ (SPORT)

Figure 3-7. Example of a medical release form.

Athletic Insurance Selection Form

Jeff's School Board, its employees, agents, and insurers, have no liability, and accept no liability for injuries or accidents occurring to students during their participation in interscholastic athletics or sports and related extra-curricular teams or activities. The student and parent(s)/guardian(s) assume any and all risks, including without limitation risk of incurring medical expenses associated with the participation by the student.

Student's Name_____ Grade_____
    (Print)

_____ We have received an insurance packet from a Jeff's School Board employee, and do not wish to purchase any such insurance, and do hereby affirm our agreement to be responsible for providing insurance covering injuries to the undersigned student athlete.

_____We have received an insurance packet from a Jeff's School Board employee, and have purchased said insurance, and proof of said purchase is attached.

Parent's Signature_____Date_____

Student's Signature _____ Date_____

Figure 3-8. Example of a health insurance information form.

ing information that may contain confidential information, it is necessary to completely fill out a cover sheet with all of the sender's information and a confidentiality statement. Although the intended receiver may be awaiting the fax, you cannot guarantee its transmission without error. The cover sheet should state who is sending the fax, the exclusive recipient, the purpose of the fax, and a confidentiality statement. The confidentiality statement should read something similar to the one listed below:

> CONFIDENTIALITY NOTICE: The material included in this facsimile transmission is intended solely for the use of the designated recipient. This communication may contain information that is confidential or privileged. Confidentiality and privilege are not lost by this fax having been sent to the wrong person. If you are not the designated recipient or the person responsible for delivering it to the designated recipient, please notify the sender immediately at the number given above. Distribution, photocopying, or use of this communication by anyone other than the intended recipient is expressly prohibited.

Be brief yet informational. Brevity and clarity are key components to designing and utilizing various documentation styles.

HEALTH INSURANCE INFORMATION

All athletes should have health insurance information on file (Figure 3-8). When an athlete is going to a medical facility other than the athletic training room, an information sheet should be sent with the athlete. The insurance information sheet should include the athlete's name, date of birth, social security number, contact information, and all insurance information, including the provider's name and policy number (see Appendix F for examples of insurance forms). It is also helpful if there is a phone number where the insurance company can be reached if a problem or question arises.

If the institution or facility is the primary or secondary provider, a copy of the institution's insurance should be sent with the individual's insurance depending on the type of payment arrangement the institution has made for its medical bills. Most institutions today are using the athlete's insurance as the primary source of payment and the institution's insurance as a secondary means of payment.

Informed Consent

The informed consent is a form that an athlete must sign stating that they understand what they are going to be participating in and the risks associated with it. The

---

Common Mistake #1

Writing editorial comments that are not part of a medical file

Suggestion for avoidance: Keep all portions of documentation factual and document in the appropriate locations. Avoid personal opinions.

Common Mistake #2

Omission of important information in a medical record

Suggestion for avoidance: Pay careful attention to documenting all pertinent medical records as soon as you can following an encounter. The longer you wait, the more likely you are to forget something that should be documented.

Common Mistake #3

Not updating medical record forms

Suggestion for Avoidance: Frequently reviewing forms to assess their accuracy and timeliness avoids using outdated documentation forms.

---

informed consent may also be referred to as a shared responsibility for sports safety (see Appendix G for examples of consent forms). The form the athlete signs outlines their knowledge that participating in sports requires an acceptance of risk. By signing the informed consent, the athlete agrees to rightfully assume that those responsible for the conduct of the sport have taken reasonable precaution to minimize such risks and that neither they nor their peers participating in sports will intentionally or knowingly inflict injury upon anyone including himself or herself.

The form usually includes an assumption of risk clause in the last paragraph. An example of a statement that may be included in this document is listed below:

> Although we often rely on officials, coaches, administration, athletic trainers, and others to legislate the rules and provide effective and proper equipment, seldom is it sufficient for them to ensure compliance of the rules and safety guidelines alone. Compliance means respect on everyone's part for the intent and purpose of a rule and/or guidelines. By signing below, I have read the shared responsibility and informed consent statement. I fully understand without question that there are certain inherent risks involved in participation in athletics. I acknowledge that these risks can and may occur and I am willing to assume responsibility for such risks while participating in athletics.

This form must be signed by all athletes. If the athlete is under the age of 18, a parent or legal guardian must sign the form as well. It is also a good idea to have a witness sign the form for validation purposes.

Pain Scales

A good way to determine the level of pain or type of pain an athlete is experiencing is to utilize pain scales. A variety of scales can be used but having a printed scale that the athlete can see when evaluating pain helps to assess what type of pain they have. Examples of pain scales that have been universally accepted among health care providers include a visual analog scale:

---

0   1   2   3   4   5   6   7   8   9   10

SUMMARY

There are numerous forms that exist that are essential in the documentation of athletic training related information. These forms range from being collective in nature to informative and communicative, acknowledging awareness and providing consent. Regardless, all forms are considered legal documents once utilized and recorded with patient information. While the process of accumulating various forms for documentation may appear to be a tedious and time consuming process, thorough and accurate documentation provides for a greater opportunity for effective care and reduces the risk of assumed liability for an athletic trainer.

DISCUSSION ITEMS

Using the information presented in this chapter, answer the following:

1. What forms do you think have been designed in your athletic training room that serve the most use with respect to a person's medical history? What about with respect to the progress of an athlete undergoing treatment for an injury?

2. Take some time to review all the documents in your athletic training room. Do any of these documents seem outdated? Do you have suggestions to revise the documents to make them more accurate and reflective of their true intentions?

3. Is your athletic training room missing any critical documents? If so, which ones?

4. How are your supervising athletic trainers informing coaches of injury updates? Is this being done in an efficient and appropriately private manner? Do you think there is a better way this can be done at your school?

Konin JG, Frederick MA. *Documentation for Athletic Training.* Thorofare, NJ: SLACK Incorporated; 2005.

Chapter 4

STYLES OF WRITING

LEARNING OBJECTIVES

Following the completion of this chapter, the reader will be able to:

1. Become familiar with the different styles of note writing.
2. Recognize the advantages and disadvantages of each style of writing.
3. Have the opportunity to implement different styles of writing.

INTRODUCTION

Just as there are many forms utilized to document one's medical record, so too are there numerous styles of writing. The most common part of a medical record that entertains a variety of writing styles is the daily treatment note. The decision for choosing a writing style may be based upon the type of setting one is in and the preference of the practitioner, among other considerations. Settings that tend to follow many of the same procedural approaches may use more standardized predeveloped forms for writing notes. This provides for a reduction in the amount of replication of documentation. Likewise, standardized forms are often helpful for larger staffs so that written communication amongst staff members can be made easier to interpret due to the familiarity with documents and terms used in them.[1]

> Always keep a notepad and something to write with handy so that you can jot down important tidbits of information.

The era of information and the increased amount of litigation related to athletics and health care have placed an emphasis on the completeness of medical documentation. Providing thorough and timely written documentation has become a time-consuming task, yet an ever-increasing responsibility of the athletic trainer. In an environment where injuries occur spontaneously and decisions must be made promptly, the task of documenting occurrences is challenging. Oftentimes, a less than optimal setting alters the way appropriate documentation should occur. Regardless, clear, concise, and complete documentation should be the goal for every encounter.

> Become familiar with all writing styles so that you can interpret the notes of other health care professionals.

WRITING STYLES

There are a number of writing styles that are formally recognized by medical and allied health care communities. Each style has its inherent strengths and weaknesses, lending to clinician and facility-based decisions regarding what style is best to use. The following writing styles are explained to provide you with opportunities from which to choose.

SOAP

The Subjective, Objective, Assessment, Plan (SOAP) note has been a standard accepted form of documentation for many years.[2-5] Its simplicity and itemized format allow both those writing notes and those reading them to quickly locate vital information. The nature of how a SOAP note is utilized has been referred to as a "problem-oriented" style of writing.[6]

Subjective

The subjective component of the SOAP note essentially tells the beginning of the story for each encounter or episode of a patient. Some refer to it as the history section of a note. Information placed here includes what patients or others share with you regarding what they saw, heard, how they feel, and other pieces of information. Often, a person will describe a series of events that took place, or one will recall a mechanism of injury. At times, one will describe a set of signs or symptoms, or chief complaints, associated with the injury or illness that is currently being evaluated. Reports of how symptoms have changed since the last encounter are also listed in this part of the note. Examples of statements that might be found in the subjective section of the SOAP note are as follows:

- The athlete complains of left knee pain since yesterday.
- No change in symptoms reported since the last treatment session.
- The coach states that the athlete has looked tired during practice.
- The athlete's parents are concerned about the upcoming surgery.

- The patient states she is improving with rehabilitation.
- The patient complains of increased soreness in his low back following the previous treatment session.
- The athlete believes that the ultrasound has benefited her injury.

Note that these statements are written in a manner to demonstrate the type of information that would be found in the subjective section. In an actual note, some of the terms listed would be appropriately abbreviated for brevity.

> Always document in an unbiased, strictly factual manner.

Objective

The objective component of the note is used as a location to place all measurable recordings and observed interventions. This section should contain unbiased opinions, observations, or facts. Measurements such as range of motion, muscle strength, muscle-girth and pain scales are all recorded in the objective section. All treatments performed on a person are also documented in this area. This not only includes the type of modality one may use, but also the specific body location and the parameters of the modality. Specific exercises performed and the number of sets and repetitions should also be included in the objective section. How a person is positioned during measurements and/or exercises should be noted in the objective section for purposes of reliability. Examples of statements that might be found in the objective section of the SOAP note are as follows:

- Range of motion for the left knee is 0 to 140 degrees.
- Pain is reported on a scale of 4/10.
- Ultrasound was performed to the right knee infrapatellar tendon area for 7 minutes at 1.4 cm² on a continuous mode at 3 MHz.
- The athlete performed 3 sets of 10 repetitions of bilateral straight leg raises with 3 pounds of resistance.
- The patient received grade III inferior glide joint mobilizations to the left glenohumeral joint in a supine position.

Again, these are examples of the type of content documented in the objective portion of the SOAP note. Many of these examples would be written slightly differently for brevity.

Assesment

The assessment component of the SOAP note serves as the location for the clinician to document his/her professional opinion regarding the patient's status. This includes an interpretation of how a patient responded to a treatment intervention, if his/her status has improved or progressed over a period of time, or even whether or not certain treatment interventions seem to be effective. Examples of how one might document a professional opinion are as follows:

- The athlete appears to be progressing with rehabilitation as straight leg raises have increased in sets, repetitions, and resistance.
- In my professional opinion, the patient has shown progress with ambulation.
- The athlete appears to be running with less pain as her reported pain has decreased from 8/10 to 4/10 in the   past week.
- The athlete should be able to begin full weight bearing in 3 to 5 days.
- The athlete appeared to have some discomfort with the administration of ultrasound.

The assessment component of the SOAP note also contains the goals that are set forth with respect to any treatment plan. Often, both short- and long-term goals are established upon the initial evaluation of a person. The recording of a patient's goal is most appropriately placed on the assessment section. These goals should include both a temporal and a measurable component. That is, the ability to measure the goal must be accomplished in some objective manner, and it needs to be done within a designated timeframe. As such, any professional opinion related to the progress, obtainment, or digression from pre-established goals is noted in the assessment area of the note. These goals should be established from a list of problems identified as they pertain to the patient or athlete. The following are content-based examples of problems and short-term and long-term goals:

Problem List

- The athlete is unable to throw a baseball 90 feet without pain and discomfort.
- The patient has significant pain in the right ankle at rest.
- The athlete has limited left shoulder external rotation.
- The athlete has weakness with right elbow flexion.

Short-Term Goals

- The athlete will be able to throw the baseball 90 feet, for 20 throws, with pain no greater than 4/10 within 2 to 3 weeks.
- The patient will achieve a reduction of pain from 8/10 to 4/10 in the right ankle at rest in 1 week.
- The athlete will gain 20 degrees of left shoulder external rotation in 2 weeks.
- The athlete will increase right elbow flexion strength from 3/5 to 4/5 in 3 weeks.

Long-Term Goals

- The athlete will be able to throw the baseball 90 feet for 50 throws pain-free within 5 to 6 weeks.
- The patient will achieve a reduction of pain from 8/10 to 0/10 in the right ankle at rest in 3 to 4 weeks.
- The athlete will gain 90 degrees of left shoulder external rotation in 6 to 8 weeks.
- The athlete will increase right elbow flexion strength from 4/5 to 5/5 in 6 weeks.

> Professional assessments should always be based on previously documented observations and measurements, as well as scientific evidence and support.

Plan

The plan is the final portion of the SOAP note, where the future approach to care is documented. The plan is based upon the cumulative findings of the subjective, objective, and assessment information, and can be determined from the most recent treatment or as a result of a number of treatment interventions. The plan is a carefully thought-out approach to determining what the next best step is for a patient or athlete. The plan should pay particular attention to the problems that need to be addressed. Examples of written statements that would be found in the plan section include the following:

- We will reduce the intensity for the next treatment session and monitor the response.
- Plan for this week is to gradually increase the amount of resistance for left knee extension exercises as tolerated by the athlete in increments of 1 pound per treatment session.
- Begin a functional running program with straight line running and right angle turns at 50% of full effort.
- Continue to administer cross-friction massage to the left biceps long head tendon on a daily basis for 1 more week.

The advantages of using the SOAP note format include following a standard and logical format each time, the ability to implement appropriate medical abbreviations within the note, the speed at which a thorough note can be completed, and the ability for clinicians to rapidly orient themselves with other clinician's notes. Though SOAP notes are written in abbreviated formats, patients or athletes with complex medical conditions or considerable intervention can make a SOAP note somewhat lengthy in general for the sake of completeness.

> Set all goals so that they are measurable and realistic.

The major disadvantage of using a SOAP note format for medical documentation includes the necessity of having all parties who will be reading the note be familiar with the style and format. Not all health care providers use the SOAP note format for various reasons, and the unfamiliarity of the documentation style may interfere with one's ability to extract vital information. Suggestions have been made to modify the standard SOAP note format to alleviate this concern.[7] Listing functional limitations (inability to run at 100%) rather than only listing impairments (knee flexion limited to 100 degrees) provides for all parties who may read a SOAP note to understand the current status of a patient. A shift toward describing functional limitations and goals seems to enhance communication among allied health care providers. The process of writing a SOAP note in a more functional format has been referred to as a functional outcome report (FOR).[8,9]

Functional outcome reporting has not only been used to assist with communication between allied health care providers, it also serves to bridge the gap for those who are not in the medical profession but are involved with reading patient medical records. Insurance company representatives, medical office personnel, and case managers would need to read and interpret medical records of clients while making critical decisions regarding the functional status of these individuals. Functional outcome reporting designed to successfully reimburse a clinician for services provided must clearly demonstrate meaningful progress as a result of treatment intervention and the ability for a person to sustain functional gains over an extended period of time, not solely when in the clinical setting.

> Demonstrate functional limitations in written documentation to more appropriately justify treatment interventions.

Narrative

A narrative style note is not so much compartmentalized because it simply tells a story in a short version format. Here, abbreviations are not typically used. Instead, complete sentences are written containing clear and concise information pertinent to the client record. Narrative note writing has advantages in medical documentation; it is a style with which all readers would be familiar. The omission of medical abbreviations makes it relatively simple for the reader regardless of his/her level of medical background or experience. The major disadvantage of using narrative writing style is that it requires a reader to search for any specifically desired information throughout the entire note. The lack of categorizing components removes the standardization of the location in which information can be found. Thus, a longer narrative note increases the difficulty of quickly locating specific pieces of information and potentially reduces the likelihood of

someone reading an entire note if the information sought can be retrieved in a quicker manner. Another disadvantage of a long narrative is that a reader may unintentionally not see important information pertaining to a patient's status. An example of a narrative style note is as follows:

The athlete has decreased pain today even though he has just run 7 miles at a moderate pace. He was treated with moist hot packs and a gentle massage to his left hamstring muscle group prior to the run, received stretching to the same muscle group after the run, followed by some ice for 15 minutes. He was instructed to continue stretching on his own and increase his mileage and intensity the next time he runs by about 10%. We will see how he feels after his next run and determine if he is ready to return to full participation with the team.

Problem-Oriented

A problem-oriented style of note writing is also seen when an individual is being treated by a number of different disciplines that all are working together to achieve a common goal. This is most commonly seen in a hospital or clinic-based setting where providers with different health care backgrounds and credentials approach a similar problem and goal with a slightly different viewpoint. For example:

A 21-year-old female lacrosse player who recently sustained a quadriceps injury may be receiving treatment from the athletic training staff with the goals of reducing pain, reducing localized inflammation, and maintaining strength in the muscle group. Simultaneously, this athlete may be working with the strength and conditioning staff, who, knowing that this individual is seeing limited playing due to the injury, may also want to focus on maintaining appropriate quadriceps strength. The ability for both the athletic trainer and the strength and conditioning coach to communicate in a manner that provides for efficient and safe treatment in an attempt to achieve a common goal of maintaining appropriate quadriceps strength can be obtained if medical records are shared and viewed by both parties. Each party can document their role in the process, being careful not to prematurely fatigue this athlete when working on the same muscle group under both disciplines. Electronic documentation whereby all parties are connected to the medical record alleviates such concerns and essentially serves as a form of problem-oriented documentation if the goals are shared in a team-like manner. The key to successful problem-oriented documentation styles is an identification and understanding of the problems and the goals by all disciplines involved. Some have expanded upon the depths of problem-oriented styles and developed what is now referred to as hypothesis-oriented, including more disability-based documentation and an inclusion of preventive care plans.[10]

Name:			Sport:		
Date	Impairment	Disability	Intervention	Outcome	Clinician

Figure 4-1. Example of a focus chart.

Anecdotal

Anecdotal documentation style essentially involves the use of preprinted forms.[11] Many clinicians will incorporate custom designed forms that meet needs of their clinical environment. This approach tends to cut down on repetitive documentation. For example, if a given facility commonly treats athletes with shoulder injuries, a predesigned form that encompasses all of the relevant information to be assessed can be utilized so that the clinician need only fill in the blanks. These forms can be handy, though they can also be time-consuming to create. Furthermore, each form should be designed in such a way that allows for any additional information relevant to the individual's condition but not specifically addressed on the given form. In addition to the time it takes to develop a standardized pre-established form, the cost of printing numerous forms must also be considered. A facility that opts for anecdotal style note writing will need to consider the many different types of forms needed to cover all of the potential documentation opportunities and needs. Throughout this text you will be introduced to anecdotal forms of documentation ranging from initial evaluation to preparticipation forms.

Focus Charting

Focus charting is a method of medical documentation that is similar to how a SOAP note is designed, with respect to categorizing subheadings. A focus chart, however, is designed in a chart-like format with relatively few important categories. Like all other forms of notation, dates and signatures must accompany written documentation. Beyond that, clinicians can opt for creating their own personal preference for categories. Figure 4-1 is an example of a focus chart derived from the terminology of Nagi's

model of disability.[12] Focus charting can be advantageous; it simplifies by category what one might be looking for in terms of obtaining quick information. This works especially well with customized categories favorable to a clinician. Limiting the size of the chart, however, may at times deter one from thoroughly completing medical records simply due to space.

Charting by Exception

Charting by exception is the most simplistic method of written documentation. With this form of note taking, only changes from previous interactions are entered into the medical record. This method does not involve detailed documentation and can utilize abbreviations or full sentences, but it typically does not elaborate on repetitive information. Often a sentence or two that summarizes each interaction is all that is included. The advantages of charting by exception are obviously that minimal time is needed to record pertinent information. Though this form of medical documentation has been used fairly liberally by some clinicians, it is the disadvantages of the style that prevent many from using it on a regular basis. The omission of information as a result of quick and minimal recording of notes has the tendency of not allowing for a thorough medical record. In a chart by exception, it is assumed that if something is not documented then there is no change from a previous patient encounter. However, not having on record a more complete picture of an interaction poses challenges to other readers when attempting to access specific medical information. Furthermore, as the medical record is considered a legal document, charting by exception contains the least amount of information provided for one to refer to when analyzing a patent's medical record for liability purposes.

Common Mistake #1

Not writing pertinent and critical information in a patient's record

Suggestion for avoidance: Document as much as you can and feel is important as soon as you can. Waiting for a period of time following an interaction with a patient increases the likelihood of forgetting important information.

Common Mistake #2

Writing notes that are ineligible

Suggestion for avoidance: Write slowly so that any party who needs access to a patient's record can read all parts of the written record.

Common Mistake #3

Using a style of writing that does not best fit your facility

Suggestion for avoidance: Analyze the forms you currently use and compare them to the type of patient interactions you have. Choose the style of writing that is most conducive to your working environment.

Common Mistake #4

Getting too comfortable and lackadaisical in note writing

Suggestion for avoidance: Periodically review notes and locate common mistakes so that they can be avoided with future written submissions into the medical charts.

REFERENCES

1. Arrigo C. Clinical documentation. In: Konin JG, ed. *Clinical Athletic Training.* Thorofare, NJ: SLACK Incorporated; 1997.

2. Kettenbach G. *Writing SOAP Notes.* Philadelphia: FA Davis Publishers; 1990.

3. *Managing Risk Through Quality PA Practice: A Guide For Health Care Providers.* Alexandria, Va: American Academy of Physician Assistants; 1994.

4. Rankin JM, Ingersoll C. *Athletic Training Management Concepts and Applications.* St. Louis, Mo: Mosby Publishing; 1995.

5. Ray R. *Management Strategies in Athletic Training.* Champaign, Ill: Human Kinetics Publishers; 2003.

6. Shaughnessy MK, Burnett CN. Implementation of the problem-oriented progress note in a skilled nursing facility. *Phys Ther.* 1979;59(2):160-6.

7. Abeln S. Importance of documentation to patient care reimbursement. In: Stewart D, Abeln S, eds. *Documenting Functional Outcomes in Physical Therapy.* St. Louis, Mo: Mosby Year Book; 1993.

8. Sawdon J. Documentation requirements. In: Curtis KA, ed. *The Physical Therapist's Guide to Health Care.* Thorofare, NJ: SLACK Incorporated; 1999.

9. Swanson G. Functional outcome reporting. In: Stewart D, Abelin S, eds. *Documenting Functional Outcomes in Physical Therapy.* St. Louis, Mo: Mosby Year Book; 1993.

10. Rothstein JM, Echternach JL, Riddle DL. The hypothesis-oriented algorithm for clinicians II (HOAC II): a guide for patient management. *Phys Ther.* 2003;83(5):455-70.

11. Meyer TJ. *A Guide to Evaluations "With Forms" For the Physical Therapist.* Thorofare, NJ: SLACK Incorporated; 1994.

12. Nagi SZ. Nagi's model of disability. In: Pope AM, Tarlov AR, eds. *Disability in America: Toward A National Agenda for Prevention.* Washington, DC: National Academy Press; 1991.

DISCUSSION ITEMS

Using the information presented in this chapter, answer the following:

1. What are the advantages and disadvantages of each writing style described in this chapter?

2. What do you feel is the most difficult part of the SOAP note to write? Why?

3. Why is it important to have temporal and measurable goals established as part of the treatment plan?

4. What do you think is the most accurate, thorough, and effective style of documentation for a high school athletic training setting? University or college setting? Clinic setting? Industrial setting?

Konin JG, Frederick MA. *Documentation for Athletic Training.* Thorofare, NJ: SLACK Incorporated; 2005.

Chapter 5

LEGAL CONSIDERATIONS IN DOCUMENTATION

LEARNING OBJECTIVES

Following the completion of this chapter, the reader will be able to:

1. Recognize the importance of careful and thorough documentation.
2. Identify the relationship between thorough documentation and liability.
3. Become familiar with privacy and confidentiality issues as they pertain to medical documentation.
4. Be introduced to methods of avoiding legal pitfalls with medical documentation.

INTRODUCTION

All information pertaining to a person's medical history is considered a part of a legal record.[1] Documents considered to be part of the record may be found in hard copy or in an electronic version, all holding the same value of importance and legal status. The compilation and accumulation of a person's medical record has been referred to as the "history" of an organization.[2] That is, all of the information demonstrates a timeline of interaction between a facility and/or provider and a patient. This history is not limited to the specific documentation of an individual, as it also includes facility and organizational documents that pertain to such items as policy and procedure, position statements, and continuous quality of care.[3-6]

Furthermore, a chronology of care can be outlined and reviewed via medical documentation.[7]

Many styles of writing and numerous forms exist as methods for properly documenting all aspects of a medical record. While no one perfect way exists to keep track of appropriate information, health care professionals understand the importance of good documentation and therefore make efforts to abide by minimal standards. While individual health care professionals can establish suggested guidelines for proper documentation, the practicality and ability to enforce required guidelines is not feasible.[8] However, there are certain components of medical record keeping that accrediting organizational bodies may require. For example, signed patient confidentiality forms and/or consent to release medical records are required for all patients regardless of the type of health care provider overseeing a service. Though standard forms may not exist for this type of information, essential components such as signatures, dates, and phrases that clearly explain the intent of a document must be included.[9] Often it is a violation of a standard of care, that can best be identified through documentation trails, that lends itself to a malpractice suit against a practitioner.

Establishing Baseline Information

In a medical record, historical information is obtained as a means to initiate a patient's medical chart. This information includes a person's biographical data, such as general and emergency contact information. Preseason preparticipation examinations and initial evaluations from injury and illness also serve as a baseline for information with respect to a person's condition. The importance of establishing baseline information cannot be underestimated. With respect to contact information, baseline information serves as the primary means for enhancing communication. In an emergency circumstance, such data are critical and timely. Data that relate to known allergies or insurance coverage become extremely valuable under emergency situations.

Baseline data obtained from physical examinations and initial injury evaluations serve as a means for measuring change over time. Having this information documented facilitates the development of measurable goals, and allows one to monitor the progression of care to assess for quality outcomes.

The development of a departmental policy and procedure manual also serves as a document where established information can be found.[3, 10,11] This serves as a blueprint for rules and regulations of how one's operation will run. Having such a document sets standards to be followed and guides staff members and students alike with respect to various circumstances. While having a plan for policy and procedure can be advantageous and serve as a proactive document, not following established policy and procedure poses great risk to those who choose to act on their own. Should one be faced with litigation, one of the first things that will be reviewed by all parties is the policy and procedures that have been established to determine whether or not one acted within the set standards.

CONFIDENTIALITY AND PRIVACY

An essential responsibility of any health care provider is to respect the privacy and confidentiality of all patients. The athletic trainer is in a position of trust, and is privy to

a significant amount of information that pertains to the health status of an athlete or patient. This information is the property of the athlete/patient. As such, each person under one's care needs to acknowledge, in written permission, a clear understanding of how medical record information will be handled and managed. This written permission should clearly spell out and explain the parameters of who has access to such information and the circumstances for which access to information will be allowed.

> Share your policy and procedures regarding the privacy and confidentiality of all athletes with coaches and media prior to incidents where information is sought.

Standard forms that detail consent to release information can be established to protect the privacy and confidentiality of patients. However, it is important for the athletic trainer to recognize that information can be shared most easily through verbal communication. Casual, nonchalant discussion often leads to accidental sharing of information that should be kept confidential. Regardless of whether information is shared in writing via the copying and transferring of medical records, or through verbal communication in an office discussion, permission must be granted appropriately. It is commonplace for staff to seek consultation from each other on given cases and incidents. Staff may want to share information with athletic training students as a learning opportunity. Such plans to share information in a professional manner should be conveyed from the onset as part of the written consent form. Otherwise, permission to seek consultation involving the sharing of confidential information must be obtained on a case-by-case basis. In cases where personal and specific consent was not provided or agreed to, generic information that omits the obvious identification of the patient/athlete can be shared for the sole purposes of seeking consultation and advice.

In 1996, the United States federal government passed a law referred to as the Health Insurance Portability and Accountability Act (HIPAA). This act, which took effect on April 14, 2003, was specifically designed to protect patients' medical records and other health information provided to health plans, doctors, hospitals, and other health care providers. The regulations in this act establish national standards for the protection of patients' medical information and specifically involve the following areas:[12]

- Access to Medical Records—Health care providers must grant a patient access to his/her own medical record upon request within 30 days time.
- Notice of Privacy Practices—Health care providers must inform all patients how they plan to use and

restrict personal medical information. As stated previously, in the athletic training settings this is often done by way of a medical records release form.

- Limits on Use of Personal Medical Information—Health care providers are not allowed to disclose personal information to any party unless previous written consent was authorized and the sharing of information relates directly to medical purposes. Athletic trainers' discussions with media are good examples of sharing information that could potentially be unauthorized to a party that has no direct bearing on the care of the athlete or patient.

- Prohibition on Marketing—This component prevents athletic trainers and all other health care providers from using any patient/athlete and their medical condition or treatment for marketing purposes without written consent.

- Confidential Communications—Regardless of what type of standardized documentation forms a facility or provider develops, patients have the right to request how and to whom they want all communications to go through.

Under HIPAA, those who must comply with regulations are referred to as "covered entities." A covered entity is defined as one of the following: a health care provider that conducts certain transactions in electronic form, a health care clearinghouse, or a health plan. The Centers for Medicare and Medicaid Services within the Health and Human Services branch of the federal government have established guidelines for determining who qualifies as a covered entity. The location for this Web site can be found in this chapter's list of references. Even though many athletic trainers may be working in facilities that are not determined to be covered entities under HIPAA, it is prudent to implement and adhere to the best actions that will protect a patient/athlete's privacy regarding medical information.

> Invest in a paper shredder so that when confidential documents can be appropriately discarded they will not be accessible by third parties.

SPECIAL CONSIDERATION FOR LEGAL DOCUMENTATION

All athletic trainers should pay particular attention to policies and guidelines that have been set by national governing and organizing bodies. Of course, state laws take precedent in all settings and should be followed by every athletic trainer regardless of setting. Organizations such as the National Athletic Trainers' Association (NATA) and the National Collegiate Athletic Association (NCAA) have developed consensus statements on a number of sports medicine related topics.[13,14] Though these positions taken by the associations are not recognized formally by any state or federal law, they do serve as the industry's suggested guidelines, and therefore would be the document to which legal authorities refer when reviewing the actions taken by an athletic trainer. Collegiate athletic training rooms are often involved with athletes who need various medications prescribed and administered by medical doctors. A university must follow all state and federal regulations and guidelines for such prescribing, dispensing, and storing of medications to athletes. While this is commonplace in university settings, it has been reported that not all institutions' policies and procedures are regularly in compliance with state and federal regulations.[15]

In many athletic training settings physicians often provide verbal orders to athletic trainers regarding the status or progression of an athlete or patient. In such cases, the athletic trainer must pay special attention to document all verbal orders like any other piece of relevant information. This is critical not only to allow for a complete and accurate medical records to which subsequent providers can relate, but also to protect the athletic trainer from potential accusations of practicing without the direction of a medical doctor.

> Make it a point to become professional associates with your facility's legal counsel.

Informed Consent

Prior to the administration of any clinical intervention, athletic trainers must obtain informed consent from all patients and athletes. This means that anyone who will be receiving care must clearly know what type of care is being rendered, the benefits and risks associated with the care provided, and alternatives for care; and they must ultimately agree to allow for such care to be rendered.[16] This is most often done in writing, including the signature of the patient and a witness, and is dated by all parties. It should be emphasized, however, that requirements for appropriate and legal binding consent might vary from state to state.[11]

Informed consent also requires the following circumstances as described by Scott[11] and Herbert[3]:

- Consent by a competent adult

- Consent by a parent/legal guardian as the surrogate decision maker when the adult patient/client is not competent or when the patient/client is a minor

- The patient's acknowledgement of understanding and consent before the intervention/treatment proceeds

- Consent is provided voluntarily and not under any mistake of fact or duress

In the athletic training setting, general informed consent is often adhered to from the onset of care and may only generically require a patient/athlete to agree to all treatments rendered regardless of what injury or illness arises. This is typically done in this manner since there is such a higher percentage of injury and illness with those participating in sports and those who are physically active that one would be encumbered in paperwork each time a potential injury or illness was evaluated and treated. It is important, therefore, for that athletic trainer to have excellent communication with those who are being treated so that clear and specific information can be provided on any given basis, including educating the patient/athlete with respect to individual circumstances involving an injury or illness that will be treated.

It may be difficult to enforce informed consent in the athletic training setting. In such circumstances, athletic trainers may abide by what is known as the emergency doctrine.[11] The emergency doctrine simply states that in circumstances where a patient is incapacitated, unable to receive disclosure information, and unable to provide informed consent, and given that the situation poses a potential life-threatening state, then the athletic trainer is not obligated to obtain informed consent to treat and intervene. There are exceptions to this, and therefore it is highly recommended that each athletic trainer consults with his/her own counsel to develop a policy on this matter.

> A good rapport with your patients and athletes may be equally as important as thorough documentation.

Legal Claims

The documentation that is established when an athletic trainer needs to respond to a legal claim is not done once served with a notice of litigation. Rather, all of the documentation previously completed constitutes the legal medical record. Thus, athletic trainers should consider during every written entry how the entry itself would hold up in a court of law. That is the standard, and that is what attorneys and expert witnesses will critically review. Thorough and complete note taking is advocated at all times and considered both professional and proactive.[17] Possessing familiarized and standardized abbreviations and forms will assist in the gathering of documents for any legal purposes.

There are no "set" lists of standardized medically accepted abbreviations. Rather, there is a long list of abbreviations that have been widely used among health care professions. Appendix B in this book includes those abbreviations that have been documented in reference textbooks on more than one occasion. Independently generated abbreviations that have been uniquely found in some facilities are not included. The more commonplace an abbreviation, the more likely it is to be accepted and understood by all health care providers and any others who read medical records.

There are some abbreviations that tend to lend themselves to simple shorthand versions of the original word. For example, "abd" is an accepted abbreviation for "abduction." There are others, however, that may be more confusing and require memorization on the part of the health care provider. "Treatment" has been written as "Rx," an example of an abbreviation without simple shorthand. Some words or terms do not have commonly accepted and published abbreviations. Two examples of this are the words "athlete" and "pain." The authors of this text propose "ath" be used for "athlete" and "p+" and "p-" be used to describe pain or absence of pain in a medical record. These proposed abbreviations have been included in Appendix B.

> Don't fall for localized medical terminology. Use only standardized accepted terms and abbreviations.

Avoiding Legal Pitfalls

In the profession of athletic training, one expects to work with individuals who are at risk of injury by the very nature of the activities in which they participate. Whether it be a high level competitive sport or a recreational activity, injuries are bound to occur. Not all injuries are handled appropriately and not all injuries heal optimally regardless of the level of care. Knowing this, persons in the profession of athletic training should take extra precaution to act appropriately in all situations and abide by laws, policies and procedures, and guidelines established for all circumstances. Furthermore, a number of steps can be taken to avoid potential lawsuits by simply acting prudently and using common sense.[18]

All entries that become part of a person's medical record should contain only factual and unbiased information. Improper entries that do not speak to objective data are not only unethical but also illegal.[8,18] A lack of detail, including abbreviated terms or words that are not universally accepted, may come across as sloppy documentation. Some may perceive it as being misinformed or uneducated with respect to professional documentation guidelines, and this perception will be used against a practitioner to attempt to correlate documentation pitfalls to clinical decision-making errors. In addition, inadequate or incomplete documentation exposes one to risk.[1] Not being able to read handwritten notes can also be problematic. It is not an acceptable defense to state that the person who wrote a note is the only one who can interpret the handwriting. All pieces of a medical record must be legible to be acceptable. Not being able to read something in a record is similar to not having the information in the record at all.

Thoroughness in documentation has been emphasized throughout this text. Perhaps one of the greatest risks to exposed liability is not what a written record contains, but rather what is omitted from the medical record.[1] A lack of information can be translated to a measurement not taken, a test not performed, a treatment intervention not provided, or a plan not thought out. In most athletic training environments, time is of the essence and athletic trainers tend to make judgments and intervene within seconds. Many times one is in a field environment with challenges posed to the ability to properly and thoroughly document. Possessing a pen and small notepad may be helpful to take shorthand notes that can be transferred after a field session to a permanent record. Electronic hand-held devices can be used in mobile settings, but they still require attention to detail with data input regardless of the convenience of having them available.

Verbal communication has been mentioned as part of a person's medical record and information. Previously, it was discussed that improper discussions without obtained permission, consent, and authorization are considered to be a legal violation of medical privacy rights. Similarly, establishing a good rapport with all those with whom you come in contact may reduce the chances of finding yourself in a liable situation.[11,19] Avoiding confrontational situations and instead making every effort to provide a sense of comfort to all those you care for demonstrates caring on your part as a health care provider. At times, this may be difficult, as the role of an athletic trainer is many, ranging from providing health care to the physically active to administrating policy and procedure to meeting the demands of coaches. Consistent behavior that analyzes situations from all points of view and responds with objective, empathetic, equitable decision making is recommended.

> Become an attentive listener and note taker, and document all relevant conversations; you never know when you will need to refer back to them.

As with most aspects of athletic training, often the little things make a difference in the outcomes we achieve. The following tidbits are provided as tips for adhering to sound legal documentation:

- Write legibly on all occasions regardless of time constraints.
- Use a dark pen: it copies better.
- Be brief, yet concise and thorough, avoiding unnecessary wordage.
- Use only universally accepted medical terms and abbreviations.
- Write on every line, not skipping or leaving blank spaces.
- Be sure to sign and date every entry in a medical record.
- Correct all mistakes in an appropriate manner, initial and date if necessary.
- Never backdate entries, instead use addendums to the record.
- Always be objective, never insert opinions or feelings.
- Be sure to document relevant phone conversations.
- Document things not done when the need to justify exists.
- Have others proofread your notes and accept feedback and criticism.
- Review others' notes and borrow examples of good writing.

> Develop and regularly review all of your documents to assure they are providing you the most current and accurate information, both from a practical and a legal perspective.

Documentation Retention

Situations that require the viewing of medical records by legal investigators most times do not occur around the same time as the incident of question. In fact, it may be years before medical documentation is requested to be reviewed as the result of a legal suit. Maintaining medical records in a safe and secure location is essential to proper administrative record keeping. Depending upon the document, guidelines may be in place that require the information to be retained for a certain period of time so the paperwork can still be accessed. Documentation retention may vary from state to state, follow federal guidelines, and be subject to institutional policies. It is incumbent upon each person who manages athletic training records to become familiar with documentation retention guidelines. Athletic trainers who utilize electronic data storage should plan to maintain a backup of the information in case hardware or software problems arise, making the information unobtainable.

Common Mistake #1

Not establishing baseline data with respect to a patient/athlete

Suggestion for avoidance: The initial evaluation, health history forms, and preparticipation physical examination each serve as key documents where critical and thorough baseline information can be obtained.

Common Mistake #2

Accidentally verbally breaching a patient's privacy

Suggestion for avoidance: Athletic trainers should treat every conversation related to the health care status of a patient/athlete as if it were private and always be aware of his/her surroundings so that confidential information is not overheard.

Common Mistake #3

Not knowing rules and regulations related to HIPAA and other patient information guidelines

Suggestion for avoidance: Athletic trainers should become familiar with all laws, rules and regulations, and policies and procedures related to confidentiality and privacy of patients' records. In-service education, staff meetings, and current professional literature all serve as good sources for learning.

Common Mistake #4

Making decisions based upon experience and instincts rather than seeking appropriate authoritative advice

Suggestion for avoidance: Athletic trainers should always refer to legal counsel when dealing with issues that pertain to the law. Though a quick response may not be provided at all times, one that is more likely to be correct serves for a better outcome.

Common Mistake #5

Not educating a patient/athlete about a therapeutic modality intervention

Suggestion for avoidance: Even though many athletes and patients alike have opportunities to observe others in clinical settings receiving therapeutic modalities (including manual therapy), they may not be aware of the risks vs. the benefits, potential adverse effects, and warning signs for harmful side effects.

Common Mistake #6

Underestimating the amount of documentation required with catastrophic events

Suggestion for avoidance: Any time a significant injury results, the athletic trainer should assume that all communications, assessments, and interventions associated with or regarding the person who has sustained the injury will ultimately be reviewed by third parties and used for further clinical and/or legal decisions.

REFERENCES

1. Feather H, Morgan N. Risk management: role of the medical record department. *Top Health Rec Manage.* 1991;12(2):40-8.

2. Harkins S. Documentation: why is it so important. *Emerg Med Serv.* 2002;31(10):89-90.

3. Herbert DL. *Legal Aspects of Sports Medicine.* 2nd ed. Canton, Ohio: PRC Publishing, Inc.; 1995.

4. Martin CA. Improving the quality of medical record documentation. *J Healthc Qual.* 1992;14(3):16-23.

5. Murphy BJ. Principles of good medical record documentation. *J Med Pract Manage.* 2001;16(5):258-60.

6. Tabak N, Ben-Or T. Legal and medical nursing aspects of documentation, recording and reporting. *Med Law.* 1995;14(3-4):275-82.

7. Cross AT. Legal requirement of private practice medical records. *J Am Diet Assoc.* 1988;10:1272-4.

8. Steffen TM, Meyer AD. Physical therapists' notes and outcomes of physical therapy. A case of insufficient evidence. *Phys Ther.* 1985;65(2):213-7.

9. Ray R. *Management Strategies in Athletic Training.* Champaign, Ill: Human Kinetics Publishers; 2003.

10. Konin JG. *Clinical Athletic Training.* Thorofare, NJ: SLACK Incorporated; 1997.

11. Scott RW. *Health Care Malpractice: A Primer on Legal Issues for Professionals.* 2nd ed. New York, NY: McGraw Hill Publishers; 1999.

12. United States Department of Health and Human Services. Protecting the Privacy of Patient's Health Information. Available at: http://www.hhs.gov/news/facts/privacy.html. Accessed January, 2004.

13. Armstrong J, Courson RW, Kleiner DM, McLoda TA. National Athletic Trainers' Association position statement: emergency planning in athletics. *J Ath Train.* 2002;37(1):99-104.

14. Binkley HM, Beckett J, Casa DJ, Kleiner DM, Plummer PE. National Athletic Trainers' Association position statement: exertional heat illness. *J Ath Train.* 2002;37(3):329-343.

15. Kahanov L, Furst D, Johnson S, Roberts J. Adherence to drug-dispensation and drug-administration laws and guidelines in collegiate athletic training rooms. *J Ath Train.* 2003;38(3):252-258.

16. King J. Consent: the patient's view—a summary of findings from a study of patients' perceptions of their consent to dental care. *Br Dent J.* 2001;191(1):36-40.

17. Ritter MA, Ritter NN. A malpractice episode: a sequence of events. *Clin Orthop.* 2003;(407):25-7.

18. Bean RV. Altering records: discrediting your best witness. *J Med Assoc Ga.* 1993;82(2):63-4.

19. Wood H. Managing malpractice liability: tips to limit your risk. *J Indiana Assoc.* 2001;80(3):12-4.

DISCUSSION ITEMS

Using the information presented in this chapter, answer the following:

1. What do you think are the key questions to ask on a preparticipation history medical intake form?

2. If an athlete were to ask you, "What is HIPAA?" how would you explain it?

3. How does HIPAA impact the various athletic training settings? Is there a difference between those athletic trainers who work in a high school setting vs. those in a clinic-based setting?

4. What would you say are the critical elements to consider when drafting a document for athletes to sign releasing their consent for you to share information regarding their medical record?

5. With your experiences thus far in athletic training clinical educational settings, what suggestions would you have for the current environment you are involved with to avoid legal risks associated with documentation errors?

6. Different rules exist regarding the retention of medical records. What are the rules at your institution? Are they institution driven? Or has state or federal government established them? Is your athletic training staff in compliance with these medical retention rules?

Konin JG, Frederick MA. *Documentation for Athletic Training*. Thorofare, NJ: SLACK Incorporated; 2005.

Chapter 6

ELECTRONIC DOCUMENTATION

LEARNING OBJECTIVES

Following the completion of this chapter, the reader will be able to:

1. Define the different types of electronic documentation available and how each can be utilized.
2. Identify the advantages and disadvantages of electronic documentation.
3. Become familiar with current and future security measures being utilized to protect electronic information.

INTRODUCTION

Imagine the following scenario taking place:

"Steve, we need to get you an ambulance to transport you to the hospital and get this leg taken care of," said Cynthia compassionately. "Let's not jump to any conclusions until we get a more thorough evaluation." It was a Friday night and they were on the 40-yard line of the city stadium. It was the 4th quarter, with 2:53 left on the clock, and the game was tied. Cynthia was the head athletic trainer for city high school and had just completed an initial evaluation of one of her players that unfortunately required further immediate attention. "The ambulance is on its way," said Bill, the assistant athletic trainer. "I contacted the hospital and sent the release code for his med-

ical records. The ambulance will have access to them as well. Steve, are your parents home?" Steve looked up from his swollen knee, "No, but they should have their videophone with them." Tapping his PDA, Bill pulled the number from Steve's records and pointed the ScreenCam at him and Steve. "Hello Mrs. Hampton. I'm here with Steve and..."

Cynthia was talking to herself and tapping her PDA, closing her connection with her office in the athletic training room as the ambulance was pulling in. "Everything's updated and the incident reports have been sent out. Wait until the risk management office sees this one. Seventh case this season on this new turf. Well maybe now they will read the report I sent."

The ambulance crew arrived a few minutes later and started their routine. "Hey Steve, I'm Christine and I am going to try and make you as comfortable as possible while we get your knee taken care of." Opening Steve's e-chart she said, "I see you are not allergic to anything and that you've never hurt this knee before. Well, first let's get an x-ray and send it off to the ER for them to take a look."

Less than a minute later: "We're sending the image over now," said Adam. He was the second emergency medical technician on the scene. He was in communication with the hospital and talking with the radiologist and physician on call.

"Well," the voice on the other end of the videophone paused. "The good news is there's no obvious fracture. However, there is a dislocation. His vital signs look good. Stabilize and transport. I'll send his e-chart to orthopedics with the scan attached." The image on the videophone went back to the registration desk as Christine began putting the porta-ray back in its case.

Cynthia was reading a listing on her PDA. "Steve, your insurance has come through with authorization for physical therapy if you need it, so I'm going to schedule you with City Physical Therapy for next week. Your parents can always change the appointments if they need to. I'll send the information to your home e-mail for you so you will have it." Steve nodded in appreciation as he was loaded onto the ambulance. As they drove off the field, Cynthia reviewed the video of Steve's injury on her PDA sent down from Coach Wilson who was filming the game. She sent a copy to Steve's e-chart and reopened the injury log for today's game…

The above demonstrated a very basic concept that the medical industry is moving toward. Though it is idealistic, there is certainly a desire to collect, record and, more importantly, exchange information more and more rapidly these days. It seems to be a driving force in the development of electronics and software as seen in the drive to manufacture cell phones and the Internet and digital cable television and the card you swipe at the checkout stand. Information is being passed from one source to another at a rate incomprehensible to most people. Eventually, it is conceivable that every piece of data about a person will be accessible electronically. Skeptics may laugh, but a look at the banking industry will show a great example of how something so farfetched can become common. Few people are able to remember a time when an ATM wasn't on every corner. In fact, because they are so common, most people are probably unaware that ATM stands for Automated Teller Machine. With the card that accesses these machines, a person is able to look at any financial information, transfer funds between accounts, make deposits, take out money, etc. However, if this were attempted 50 years ago, people would have been skeptical. There would have been a lack of trust, technology and security concerns, and a refusal to utilize the process because it wasn't familiar. Now there is direct deposit, automatic withdraw-

al, ATM machines at the checkout counter, and even tow trucks and taxicabs take Visa and MasterCard. The point is, as technology evolves and becomes widely utilized, skepticism is replaced by commonplace.

Personal medical information is in the process of becoming as widely accessible as financial information. The health care industry is aware of the benefits of electronic data over paper with regards to a substantial reduction in both the handling and processing time compared to paper, as well as the risk of lost paper documents. Inefficiencies of handling paper documents due to human error can be eliminated, significantly reducing administrative burden, improving overall data quality, and lowering operational costs. Medical data have a tremendous value in research, development, and even marketing. Knowing what medication to market to a given population and at what price range can result in millions of dollars in revenue. However, like the banking industry that had to slowly accept the electronic revolution, the medical field has its skeptics, a lack of trust, and an unwillingness to adapt to change. As electronic documentation evolves and is utilized at a greater capacity, the process of documenting electronically will become easier and more common.

Currently, medical information is recorded in written form for many reasons. The most obvious is that, as humans, we have a limited capacity to remember anything. So we are constantly searching for a better way to record information and, most importantly, retrieve and share it. Storage and retrieval of that data is at this time a cumbersome and costly process. What if, however, that same information could be stored on a volume of CDs or a hard drive instead of in a warehouse and retrieval of that information could be done at the touch of a button? Such is the electronic world.

> It is important to consider what the data collected will be used for, who needs to have access to it and for what purpose, and how much power is needed before deciding what type of program to use.

ELECTRONIC DOCUMENTATION DEFINED

Electronic documentation is a catchall phrase used to describe the process of collecting data or information with an electronic device such as a tape recorder, video camera, or computer. Currently, most health care offices will use a computer system to record patient information (name,

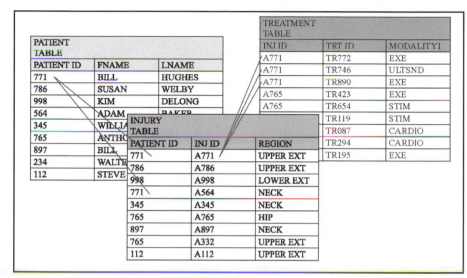

Figure 6-1. Patient information table using different fields of data.

phone, address, appointment schedule, etc.) but will keep all medical information in a paper chart or folder stored in cabinets and later archived in warehouses. Electronic documentation guidelines suggest that all patient data, including daily notes and progress notes, lab and radiology reports, and even x-ray and other diagnostic imaging, be stored digitally on a computer in a system for storage and possible retrieval.

> If there isn't a system set up to easily find and retrieve the information being recorded, then it makes little sense to record it in the first place.

Film and Video

Film and video are usually utilized as educational tools; however, pictures and videotape can be extremely valuable when included as part of a patient's medical record. The ease of taking digital photos allows one to take images that demonstrate postural changes, wound appearances, and other injury-related conditions. With video compression improving, this medium now can be stored on a computer hard drive or other data storage device. Taking videos of each patient may be easy, but it may not be the best system from the standpoint of retrieval.

Voice Recorder

Still widely utilized in the medical setting, dictating chart notes for transcribing at a later date is a common form of note taking. However, until voice recognition software is improved to the point of being a valuable tool, the information recorded still has to be manually typed into a computer, and is usually then printed for insertion into a patient's chart. With advances in technology, voice commands may some day be used to enter data. For example, selecting words in a drop down list and common commands like "tab" or "click" might be used to complete an online form.

Computers

The process of entering collected data into a computer for storage and later retrieval is relatively simple. The data can be entered in many different formats with the most popular being text documents, spreadsheets, and databases. Recent software developments have combined all of them together. With computerized documentation, the type of hardware and software compatibility must be considered.

Text Documents

This is simply entering data in paragraph format. Key words can be noted but essentially the information reads like a book or short story. This is the popular format for dictation and SOAP notes that have been stored in paper charts. Keeping this information only in digital format can be tedious because file naming can be difficult. Each file would have to be named in a way that identified the patient, the date, and the general contents of the document so that, if needed, the information could be gathered. One major drawback to the simple document is that unless an ongoing document is kept (information added to the end of the previous entry), general information like name, injury, etc would have to be repeated.

Spreadsheet

A spreadsheet is merely a simple table of columns and rows. Each column is a separate field containing specific information and each row is an individual record (Figure 6-1). This method would enable the user to sort and search for information based on individual fields.

Database

The database is a type of software designed to hold information in table format and is utilized so that the data can be stored in a logical order and retrieved in a specific yet simple fashion. The advantage of a database over a spreadsheet, or even a document creator, is that the information is not repeated and can be easily retrieved.

A database stores information in tables that are related to each other. A table consists of columns, each with a different field, and rows, each holding a separate record. For example, each field in the patient table contains information about the patients being seen (ie, names, addresses, phone numbers, etc). Each row contains an individual patient's information. The best thing about a database is it can contain more than one table, and those tables can be related to each other. An example would be the "ID" field in the patient information table. This can be a common field, meaning it will be in the injury table as well. This way the patient's information does not have to be duplicated in the injury table every time the patient is seen for a new injury. Figure 6-1 shows an example of this.

Notice that "Bill Hughes" was seen for 2 different injuries and that one of his injuries was treated 3 times. However, data never had to be duplicated because of the database system. For retrieval purposes, searching for a match in any field can collect data. For example, the "ID" field is unique to each patient, so searching for a specific one will give only 1 response—the patient being searched for. In the injury table, searching for "knee" in the "body part" field could provide many responses, as more than 1 patient could have a knee injury. The point is, information can be pulled or queried, based on the need of the person asking the questions.

Creating forms (visual documents with blank spaces for the user to fill in) with dropdown lists with responses to questions that can be clicked on speeds the process of entering data over typing. This allows the user to enter data systematically and logically that is stored automatically in the necessary tables, making the process of using complex software easier.

Regardless of how the information is stored, there are a number of factors that influence the decision regarding which system will present the greatest efficacy and benefits for its users. These include the ease of finding information quickly and efficiently, as well as costs, general ease of use, adaptability, and security.

Common Misconceptions of Electronic Documentation

Using Electronic Documentation is Always Faster and Easier

A shocking disappointment is thinking that electronic documentation will be faster and easier than paper charts. Unfortunately, this isn't entirely true. Training and data entry are extremely slow processes that need to be nurtured through the developmental stages. Additionally, the means to record data is also in the developmental stage and will evolve as users dictate what is required. Like anything else, as the user becomes more familiar with the system, the process becomes faster and easier. Fortunately, a bigger picture shows us that management of the data collected, from storage to backup to analysis, and the exchange of that data, is exponentially faster than sorting through paper charts by hand. Just be ready for that first year slow down.

The Cost is Less as There is a One Time Fee

As with anything else, there are initial startup costs associated with starting an electronic documentation system. However, maintenance, development, and mistakes can be costly. Furthermore, newer, improved, and upgraded versions of software may be associated with more fees. The computer database presents the greatest advantages with regards to retrieval, minimal duplication of data, and easy storage, although the initial costs can be a disadvantage. However, what is gained in efficiency and the ability to communicate with other entities in the health care community will more than make up for the expenditure.

> Never skimp on performance. If there is anything to learn about the evolution of the computer and software industry it is that technology moves quickly. As soon as a fast machine is developed, software developers will push it to its limits until a faster machine is built.

CURRENT CONSIDERATIONS

One advancement technology has presented is the touch screen. This allows the user to select or click on responses to predetermined questions in a software program or form by touching them on the screen, bypassing the keyboard and mouse. Items in a dropdown list or preformatted paragraphs can be easily selected, and the type of equipment is becoming easier to use and much more portable.

Another advancement is in the area of voice recognition. Still in its developmental stages, this would allow the user to enter data directly into a form or document during the evaluation by speaking into a recorder or microphone. An advantage of this is that information could be recorded into the necessary software programs as it was retrieved from the patient. No second step of typing or data entry would be required. Additionally, the equipment needed to be carried by each health care provider could be as simple as a hand held computer screen wirelessly connected to a main computer.

Currently, there are 3 main types of computer database management systems on the market. The first is a stand-alone system on a single computer or small office network. This incorporates a desktop computer and database software into which data is entered. This software can be generic like Microsoft's Access or something specifically designed for the purpose like CSMI's Sportsware (www.csmisolutions.com). Sportsware is designed in a way to record patient information in 3 main sections: demographics, injury information, and treatment log. As stated before, it is structured on a relational database platform so that data (name, address, etc) only has to be entered once, and retrieval of information is as simple as asking a question (ie, how many soccer players had ankle injuries last season?) The advantages of software programs like this is that they are relatively inexpensive and can utilize current hardware that may have more than 1 function in the office, meaning they don't require sole use of a computer or network, making the system more cost effective. When placed on a small office network, more than 1 user can enter data at a time and some can be set up to receive data previously entered on a hand held device, portable laptop, electronic notepad, or similar device. Some systems have been developed that will also function as a scheduler and can be incorporated with billing software as well. Another advantage of a system like this is that the data collected are under the control of the user. Information can be backed up, stored, and retrieved at the user's discretion. A concern with this type of system is security. Though improving with administrator passwords and levels of user accessibility, data can still be accessed and altered by unauthorized users. If installed on a network attached to the Internet, additional security measures are required to prevent unauthorized access to confidential material.

The second type of system incorporates the desktop computer with access to the Internet. The user logs onto a centralized system of computers through an Internet connection to enter data about a current patient. An example would be a program called Treat It (www.treat-it.com), which handles scheduling, and billing is driven by the health care practitioner's section of the evaluation and treatment program. With this type of program, there is an initial startup cost and usually a monthly fee for services provided. These services can include data storage, backup and retrieval, scheduling, and research and analysis for billing. The advantage is that all medical information is stored and managed offsite and the company has the resources necessary to provide up-to-date security measures to protect and back up the data. Access to the information is possible, scheduling and billing are incorporated, and the power to handle a large patient load is available with little or no startup costs for hardware and software outside of what may have been purchased for general office needs.

The third system available is the most adaptable, most powerful, and yes, most expensive to implement. This is an all-encompassing system designed to record, store, and retrieve information, as well as handle scheduling, billing, and research. It utilizes a central server computer (or network of computers) with workstations available to the health care practitioners and essential office personnel. This type of system most generally is used by large medical facilities. The software usually begins with a generic program that is then designed to meet the specific needs of the organization. An example would be building preformatted paragraphs to be inserted into a SOAP note by selecting or clicking on them in a drop down menu.

> The reason to implement an electronic documentation system is to make the processes of storage, backup, retrieval, and exchange simple, efficient, time saving, and cost effective.

Anyone with a little knowledge of how a computer works understands the concept of compatibility. For a computer to be able to open or understand a file, it needs the program installed that created the file, or the ability to convert the file to a readable format. For example, imagine if company "A" was trying to share information with company "B". Company "A" uses a document creator software to record all of its data while company "B" uses photo editing software to record all of its data. Each company would not be able to read each other's electronic data unless they had the software used to create the files. This example is what currently is happening in the health care industry. As the need for electronic data has risen, software companies and developers are working independently to try and meet that need. Unfortunately, compatibility issues have not been addressed. This problem is even greater when considering the communication needed between health care providers and health plans. One organization attempting to solve this problem is the federal government through components of HIPAA.

One section, titled The Administrative Simplification provisions of the Health Insurance Portability and Accountability Act of 1996 (HIPAA, Title II), requires the

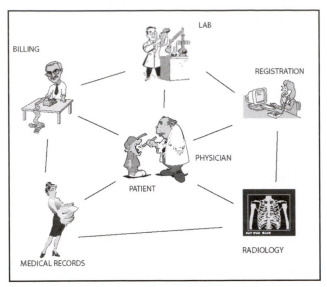

Figure 6-2. The big picture: exchange of information.

Department of Health and Human Services to establish national standards for electronic health care transactions and national identifiers for providers, health plans, and employers. It also addresses the security and privacy of health data. Adopting these standards will improve the efficiency and effectiveness of the nation's health care system by encouraging the widespread use of electronic data interchange in health care.

Differences in Athletic Training Settings

The type of athletic training setting one is in will often play a major role in determining what type of electronic software, if any, is used. Most athletic trainers employed in clinical settings have been exposed to a form of electronic documentation, either through scheduling or billing purposes. The nature of the setting, being a somewhat controlled environment, and the requirements associated with reimbursement necessitate electronic data.

High school settings may use electronic documentation systems to assist with record keeping. The ease of this is that often a single workstation can be used because only 1 athletic training room exists in most high schools. User fees for a single station keep overall long-term costs minimal. Cost is always an overriding factor in a high school setting, perhaps more so than any other setting.

Those in university or college settings have increasingly moved to electronic documentation as a result of the volume of information associated with large numbers of ath-

letes potentially spread out over a number of venues. The cost associated with such usage becomes quite high. However, managing a paper trail of data for multiple venues becomes quite difficult given the need for centralized data storage as a means of efficiency.

Athletic trainers in industrial type settings may find themselves using either paper or electronic documentation methods depending upon the nature of the industry for which they work. One who provides services for a client in the technology area might be more inclined to have a software system available that can be utilized for documentation. On the other hand, if one is employed or contracted through an agricultural firm, a paper trail might be sufficient for the administration.

Advantages of Electronic Documentation

Perhaps the most obvious advantage to electronic forms of documentation is the ease of which one can store and retrieve data. Once a person is familiar with a software program, interfacing can also be relatively user friendly. Those programs that lend themselves to wireless capabilities will enable athletic trainers to document while on the road or on the field in real time. This lends the potential to record more timely and accurate information while also retrieving valuable data in case of emergency situations. As more programs develop and more users find the necessity for electronic forms of documentation, standardized systems may be created to allow for an accumulation of data that can contribute to outcomes research.

Disadvantages of Electronic Documentation

Without a doubt, the cost of purchasing, maintaining, and upgrading both computer hardware and software is the biggest disadvantage of electronic forms of documentation. Currently, operational systems that are built with different necessities in mind deter users of various organizations to interface with one another. Until a more standardized operating system is developed and embraced, information sharing will be kept to a minimum. Furthermore, without uniform operational systems, there is a learning component associated with each system with which all users must become familiar. Athletic trainers who have been working for many years with paper forms of documentation may not find it an easy adjustment to learn the benefits and challenges associated with today's capabilities of technology.

Common Mistake #1
Assuming that using electronic software will save an athletic training program money
Suggestion for avoidance: Research the type of electronic documentation you wish to use and thoroughly assess all costs associated with purchasing, maintaining, and upgrading the program.

Common Mistake #2
Thinking that using an electronic documentation system for athlete information is always user friendly and can be implemented as soon as the program is purchased
Suggestion for avoidance: Plan ample amounts of time for software training so that all athletic trainers and other users are familiar with a system prior to the time you wish to implement it.

Common Mistake #3
Assuming all software programs are the same and compatible for all settings and all computers
Suggestion for avoidance: Incorporate the expertise of the technology staff wherever you work and ask them to review the hardware and software requirements of a documentation system that you are interested in using in your athletic training setting.

SUMMARY

Electronic forms of documentation rival all forms of information that need to be compiled in a written format. The concept of storing and retrieving data is not a new one to the health professions, yet it has only just begun to work into most athletic training environments. Figure 6-2 shows the exchange of information in a medical setting. The nature of the high volume of patient interactions on a daily basis, live on-the-field assessments, travel, and other incidental circumstances, make it a challenge for the modern day athletic trainer to adjust to an electronic system of documentation.

DISCUSSION ITEMS

Using the information presented in this chapter, answer the following:

1. What is the most advanced form of electronic documentation that you have seen used in your institution? What are its advantages and disadvantages?

2. How do you think an electronic documentation system will affect the overall profession of athletic training 10 years from now?

3. Does your school currently use an electronic documentation system for inventory? Why or why not? If yes, is the program successful?

4. What security challenges threaten the use of Web-based injury reports that athletic trainers may send to coaches on a daily basis?

5. Can you think of a use for electronic documentation that would benefit athletic trainers the most, something that you have not yet seen implemented or perhaps even heard of?

Konin JG, Frederick MA. *Documentation for Athletic Training*. Thorofare, NJ: SLACK Incorporated; 2005.

Chapter **7**

DOCUMENTATION FOR REIMBURSEMENT

LEARNING OBJECTIVES

Following the completion of this chapter, the reader will be able to:

1. Understand the elements of proper documentation for reimbursement purposes.
2. Be aware of the legal issues surrounding reimbursement.
3. Know the difference between International Classification of Diseases and Current Procedural Terminology codes.
4. Know where to find resources on reimbursement issues.

INTRODUCTION

There is one main principle to adhere to when applying for reimbursement for athletic training services: If it isn't documented, it didn't happen! The corollary to that statement is: If it didn't happen, it won't be reimbursed. There are many other barriers to reimbursement that will be encountered throughout the process, but that rule, if ignored, is insurmountable.

The purpose of this chapter is to guide the athletic training student through the mechanisms of applying for reimbursement; documentation being the key! It is a general overview since each institution or organization employing athletic trainers will have its own criteria for being paid for services rendered by the athletic trainer.

This chapter is also limited to the reimbursement process general to outpatient clinical practice. It will become obvious that there are 2 types of documentation necessary for reimbursement: documentation on patient treatment or status and documentation required by payers for payment of services. While athletic trainers are certainly employed in venues that treat workers' compensation clients or Medicare/Medicaid patients, the documentation and practice requirements of those patients are beyond the level of this chapter.

Get connected! Log on to the federal government's Web site for the Center for Medicare and Medicaid Services. Know what restrictions are placed on providers of services for patients who qualify for these benefits.

PARAMETERS AFFECTING REIMBURSEMENT

Legal Issues

The first requirement to be met by the athletic trainer is that the state wherein the athletic trainer is practicing legislatively allows the athletic trainer to bill for services rendered. In other words, the profession of athletic training must be regulated by the state and the regulatory act must allow for billing of services. The athletic trainer is responsible for knowing the law that governs his/her profession. It is not the responsibility of the employer, although the employer should be cognizant of the appropriate law to prevent asking the athletic trainer to inadvertently violate the law.

A common example of inadvertent violation of law is having a clinical athletic trainer treat a Medicare patient and then bill an intermediary for the Center for Medicare & Medicaid Services (CMS) for the services. CMS is a division of the Health and Human Services Agency (HHS) of the federal government. While athletic trainers are able to treat Medicare patients, CMS cannot be billed for the services rendered by an athletic trainer. Athletic trainers are not recognized as approved providers in the Medicare Act. Reimbursement is limited to the service given by an approved provider like a physical therapist or a physical therapy assistant under the supervision of a physical therapist. To bill CMS for services rendered by an athletic trainer, even if supervised by a physician or physical therapist, is considered Medicare fraud. The Federal Office of the Inspector General and the FBI vigorously investigate Medicare fraud, and federal courts treat violations harshly. The importance of knowing this information is that regardless of how much knowledge an athletic trainer has documenting reimbursable services, even the most accurate form of documentation may not be legal.

Another common law violation is when the athletic trainer treats an inappropriate patient. For example, in Minnesota, athletic trainers are restricted to treating patients with injuries that are related to sports participation. To have an athletic trainer treat a patient's injuries from a car accident would be a violation of the law. The athletic trainer would be liable for criminal prosecution. It can't be emphasized enough that the athletic trainer must know the law and know how the law restricts his/her practice. Common restrictions include patient class (eg, restricted to athletes), injury type (eg, resulting from participation in sports), body part injured (eg, restricted to extremities), or supervision (eg, restricted to MD, DO, or DDS). Again, documenting even the most thorough and accurate note is inappropriate in this type of a case as it reflects an illegal treatment intervention.

Third-Party Payer Requirements

The second parameter is based on the reimbursement guidelines of a third-party payer. A third-party payer is an insurance company who pays the health care provider for services rendered to an insured patient. Athletic trainers may or may not be listed on the panel of providers held by each company. Each policy offered by a company may or may not include permission to be billed for athletic training services. Depending on the restrictions determined by the purchaser, a third-party payer might have its own set of limitations regarding reimbursement. Usually, the purchaser of the policy is the employer of the athlete or his/her parents if the athlete is under the age of 25. Determining which third-party payers and even which policies offered by the payer reimburse for athletic training services is a quagmire at best. It is the responsibility of the athletic trainer's employer and the accounts receivable department to keep track of the payments or denials. However, if the athletic trainer is responsible for generating invoices to third-party payers, it is often helpful to maintain a running list of which payer paid for which services and at what rate. In doing that, the athletic trainer can forecast reimbursement trends from a payer and also has appropriate records of prior payments to use in case of denials.

Employer Requirements

The last parameter affecting reimbursements are the policies and procedures of the employer of the athletic trainer. Many health care organizations have credentialing criteria of their own that must be met before an employee may begin billing for services. It is important for an athletic trainer to ask about the credentialing process when interviewing. It may be a hardship for an athletic trainer to find out that he or she is restricted to aid duties if he/she expected to treat patients.

MECHANICS OF REIMBURSEMENT

Once a patient presents him or herself for treatment by an athletic trainer, several functions need to occur. Either the receptionist or personnel of the billing department perform many of these functions. Again, the following steps are outlined for the athletic training student should he/she become responsible for them. These steps are fully explained in a manual published by the American Medical Society (AMA) titled *Mastering the Reimbursement Process.*

> Become familiar with standardized acceptable medical abbreviations to reduce your denial rate for reimbursement.

Prescription

The primary document needed by the athletic trainer is a written prescription for evaluation and treatment from a physician. In some states, chiropractors or physical therapists, in addition to medical physicians or osteopathic physicians, are allowed to refer patients to athletic trainers by the state athletic training practice act. In some states, athletic trainers are allowed to evaluate and treat an injury for a specific period of time before seeking a prescription from a physician. However, third-party payers will not reimburse for services that are not prescribed by a physician, no matter what is written in the athletic training law.

A physician prescription must include a diagnosis, an order for evaluation and treatment, any precautions based on the diagnosis, physician's goals for the patient, and dates and signatures. It is very important to obtain the medical diagnosis from the physician. Third-party payers will compare the diagnoses entered on the billing statements from the physician's office and from the athletic training clinic. Any discrepancy will cause an automatic denial for reimbursement for the services rendered by the athletic trainer. Only physicians have the legal right to establish a diagnosis. Subsequently, payers will only recognize a physician's diagnosis. If the prescription does not include a diagnosis, contact the physician's office as soon as possible to obtain it.

Patient Registration

At the first encounter with a new patient, have the patient (or parent/guardian if the athlete is a minor) complete a registration form. Critical information that needs to be captured includes address, telephone number, brief medical history (especially presence of allergies or prior injuries), and a waiver allowing release for medical information to insurance companies and allowing payments by the insurance company to the provider. The address and telephone number is necessary should the patient need to be contacted about payments of missed appointments. Additional information could include insurance information (see below), name of referring physician and source of information about the clinic (for marketing purposes).

Insurance Information

The next document needed before treatment can be rendered is a copy of the athlete/patient's health insurance card. Photocopying both sides of the card is necessary. The card should clearly indicate the policyholder with an identification number, a group and/or policy number, an address for billing purposes, and a telephone number to call to verify accuracy of the coverage. Also, have the athlete or patient sign and date an agreement that he/she will be responsible for whatever portion of athletic training services billed that is not reimbursed by the insurance company. This document is particularly necessary should the athlete or patient not carry health insurance.

It is necessary to contact the insurance company within 24 hours, if possible, to ascertain any limitation of services. Using the policy number, the representative from the company can determine how many visits for treatment are available, in what time period the services must be provided, which services are nonreimbursable, and when physician reevaluation is necessary. In return, the company representative will ask the name and credentials of the primary provider, the type of facility where the services will be rendered, and its address and telephone number. Facilities are divided into 3 types by CMS. Most health insurance companies utilize the same system. The premise of the system is the availability of a physician to intervene in a treatment if necessary.

1. Services rendered in an inpatient facility can receive the highest reimbursement rate for similar services. However, this rate is tempered by the use of blanket payments based on the diagnosis. More frequent use of services lowers the reimbursement per treatment.

2. Services rendered in a hospital-based outpatient clinic are reimbursed on a "usual and customary rate." These rates are based on many factors, including geography and average salaries. However, services rendered in this setting are "incident to" those of a physician. Subsequently, a physician must be present within the office suite that holds the treatment facility. The services are also invoiced as part of the physician's billing statement.

3. Services rendered in an outpatient facility do not require the presence of a physician but are reimbursed at a much lower rate than found in the other types.

> Encourage your employer to spend the money each year to purchase the most updated version of the CPT and ICD-9 codes.

Ask for specific billing forms should the health insurance company require its own forms to be used. Submitting invoices on the wrong form is another common reason for denial of payment. Finally, record the name of the company representative, his/her title, and the date and time of the telephone call.

Insurance Forms

The 3 most common forms used by billing departments for invoicing payers are CMS 1500, UB 92, and HCPCS. Several years ago, the federal government tried to influence health insurance companies to accept these forms as a method of reducing health care costs. Most companies use these forms but it is necessary to inquire about them, as noted above. CMS 1500 forms are used in outpatient clinics, UB 92 forms are used in hospitals, and HCPCS forms allow for billing of supplies used in hospital procedures. We will discuss completing the CMS 1500 form.

CMS 1500 form

The CMS 1500 form is available online in Adobe format at www.cms.hhs.gov/providers/edi/cms1500.pdf. The form is a single one-sided sheet. The form is divided into numbered sections. The upper half of the form requires patient and insurance company data and is self-explanatory. The upper half of the form also requires a signature for release of medical information and allows assignment of the payment to the provider. The lower half of the form begins with line 14.

Line 14 asks for the initial date of injury
Line 15 asks for dates of similar previous injuries
Line 16 asks for dates of lost time from work
Line 17 asks for name of provider
Line 17A asks for an ID number

The federal government will require a national provider number (NPI) by May of 2005. The NPI will be required for assignment of payments in Medicare and Medicaid invoices. It remains to be seen if athletic trainers will be able to obtain an NPI from HHS since athletic trainers are not approved providers for Medicare patients. However, insurance companies have allocated provider numbers of their own to allied health personnel in order to facilitate processing of invoices. This is particularly true of prepaid organizations such as health maintenance organizations.

Line 18 asks for hospitalization dates
Line 19 is reserved
Line 20 asks for charges for an outside lab
Line 21 asks for diagnosis—this is codified in the ICD-9 Manual
Lines 22 and 23 are for Medicaid resubmission
Line 24A asks for dates of service
Line 24B asks for the code for place of service
Line 24C asks for the code for type of service

Line 24D asks for procedure—this is codified in the CPT Manual
Line 24E again asks for diagnosis and which procedures were used
Line 24F asks for charges in dollars
Line 24G asks for days or units of service and is necessary when treating a patient several times per day
Line 25 asks for a federal tax ID number—this is usually the provider's Social Security Number or the Employers Identification number
Line 26 is the patient's account number
Line 27 asks if assignment of payment is allowed
Line 28 asks for total charges in dollars
Line 29 asks for the amount paid by another payer
Line 30 is the balance of remaining charges
Lines 31, 32, and 33 ask for signature, facility address, and billing department

The form should be typed or printed and reviewed for missing information before being submitted. Any missing information is cause for immediate rejection of the claim.

> Often codes associated with billing procedures undergo changes. Be sure to familiarize yourself with the most current listings.

ICD-9 and CPT Manuals

The CMS form asked for diagnosis and procedures used on the patient. Providers and payers have codified these subjects for use. ICD-9 stands for International Classification of Diseases, 9th edition. St. Anthony's Press, among others, publishes it and it is periodically reevaluated for inclusion of new diagnoses. It consists of 3 volumes. Volume 1 is a listing of all diagnoses in a 5-digit code. Volume 2 is an alphabetical listing of all listings in the same five-digit code. Volume 3 is a listing of inpatient or in-hospital procedures. As one can see from the CMS form, having the correct diagnosis is fundamental to being reimbursed for any service provided. As indicated above, correlation of diagnosis between the physician's office and rehabilitation provider is critical to being reimbursed.

The CPT Manual stands for Current Procedural Terminology and is published annually by St. Anthony's Press and the publishing arm of the AMA. The CPT Manual contains 5-digit codes that describe procedures used in care of the patient/athlete. Use of CPT codes for reimbursement are restricted to state-regulated providers whose state law allows that the procedure be performed within the borders of the state. In other words, athletic trainers must be licensed/certified/registered by the state and the law must allow that athletic trainers can perform the procedure. One cannot claim regulation from another state as an exemption when the services are performed elsewhere. Any variance from the opinions above may leave the athletic trainer vulnerable to accusations of insurance fraud.

CPT Codes

Athletic trainers are specifically mentioned in the 97000 series of the CPT codes. The 97000 series is the Physical Medicine section. While other codes are applicable to athletic trainers (such as found in the 29000 series: casting and splinting), the vast majority of procedures used by athletic trainers in a clinical setting are found in Physical Medicine. The 97000 procedure series is divided into timed/nontimed and supervised/unsupervised procedures. Timed procedures are reimbursed in 15-minute blocks while nontimed treatments are reimbursed for the activity only. Supervised procedures require the presence of the state-regulated provider for performance of the procedure whereas an aide may monitor an unsupervised procedure. Common 97000 codes are listed below and descriptions are taken from the CPT 2002 Manual, published by the AMA.

Evaluation Codes

97005/97006 are codes for athletic trainer evaluation and reevaluation. These are nontimed codes specific to state-regulated athletic trainers.

Modalities are defined as physical agents that affect tissue.

97010 is used for hot and cold packs; in general, these modalities are no longer reimbursed.

97014 is used for unattended electrical stimulation; typically, High Volt Galvanic Stimulation or Interferential Electric Stimulation treatments would fall in this category.

97016 is used for vasopneumatic devices and is considered an unsupervised modality.

97020 is used for microwave therapy and is considered an unsupervised modality.

97022 is used for whirlpool and is considered an unsupervised modality.

97024 is used for diathermy and is considered an unsupervised modality.

97026 is used for infrared therapy and is considered an unsupervised modality.

97028 is used for ultraviolet light therapy and is considered an unsupervised modality.

97032 is used for electrical stimulation where the provider is performing one-on-one contact with the patient (supervised); trigger point therapy would fall into this category and is reimbursed in 15-minute blocks (timed).

97033 is used for iontophoresis and is considered a supervised and timed modality.

97034 is used for contrast baths and is considered a supervised and timed modality.

97035 is used for ultrasound and is considered a supervised and timed modality.

97036 is used for Hubbard tank treatments and is considered a supervised and timed modality.

97039 is used for unlisted modalities (indicate modality and time).

Procedures are defined as the skills, techniques, or services to improve function. They are considered supervised timed activities.

97110 is used for exercises to develop range of motion, strength, endurance, and flexibility.

97112 is used for exercises to improve balance, proprioception, or muscle reeducation.

97113 is used for aquatic exercises.

97116 is used for gait training.

97124 is used for massage.

97139 is used for any unlisted procedure; it requires an explanation of the procedure and the amount of time used.

97140 is used for manual therapy such as joint or soft tissue mobilization or manual traction.

97150 is used for group procedures; any time a provider treats more than 1 patient in a given time period, the group code is to be used in lieu of a specific modality or procedure code. For example, leading a group of patients through aquatic exercises or plyometric exercises would necessitate using the group code rather than 97113 or 97110.

97504 is used for fitting orthotics along with instruction in their use.

97520 is used for prosthetic training.

97530 is used for exercises to improve functional activities.

97545 is used for the first 2 hours of work hardening activities.

97546 is used for each additional hour of work hardening activity.

97750 is used for administration and evaluation of physical performance tests and measurements; a written report is required.

Here are several suggestions when using CPT Codes: (1) always use a current manual, (2) list procedures performed from major to minor, (3) use modifiers as necessary. Modifiers are 2-digit code extensions that explain extenuating circumstances in patient treatment. For example, modifier 50 is used when the procedures are performed bilaterally and modifier 59 is used when treating 2 separate injuries on the same patient in the same treatment session.

The "8 Minute Rule"

Medicare/Medicaid regulations now require that the patient not be billed for the first 8 minutes of a rehabilitation session. It is assumed by CMS that the patient is preparing for treatment and, subsequently, is not yet being treated. So, any timed modality or procedure begins being reimbursed at the 8th minute. A second timed modality or procedure cannot be billed until the 23rd minute and so on. Many insurance companies are now requiring that providers record their one-on-one time with a patient as well as the duration of any nontimed modalities. CMS has proposed, though it has not started the discovery portion of the implementation process, that providers be limited to the maximum number of timed procedure blocks for reimbursement. In other words, if a provider worked for 10 hours in a day, then the provider would be limited to billing for only 40 blocks of modalities or procedures. Obviously, nontimed procedures (like group exercise) would not qualify for this restriction but the provider could not bill for timed and nontimed activities in the same 15 minutes. Postrehabilitation note writing time is also not reimbursable.

Athletic trainers should not be overly concerned about the total time interpretation. Athletic trainers have long treated many athletes during the same time period in the athletic training room. High quality, professional care has been and is being rendered to the athletes. Group exercise or unsupervised modalities are not reimbursed at a high rate when compared to supervised and timed procedures, but an athletic trainer should be able to treat more athletes or patients in a day, should the trend come to pass.

State laws differ regarding what types of patients athletic trainers can legally treat. Know your practice act!

Denials

It is a given that many claims submitted to payers are denied immediately. Common reasons for denials include incomplete or unsigned forms, services rendered by an ineligible provider, lack of medical necessity, services considered to be "maintenance" without expectations for improvement, invoices not submitted within a specific time period, no physician prescription, or a difference in diagnosis with the referring physician's office. Unless specifically written as a clause in the payer-provider contract (particularly seen in HMOs), many providers will take 30 to 90 days to pay a "clean" invoice.

If a claim is denied, resubmit the claim as an appeal after making whatever corrections are required by the payer (some payers use their own appeal forms). Be firm in answering any assertions that indicate lack of patient progress or lack of medical need by the patient. Refer to the physician's expectations and the patient goals. Indicate whether the payer has reimbursed similar services on other patients in the past. If the appeal is also denied, be ready to ask the referring physician for assistance and to submit this appeal (with supporting literature) to the chief medical officer of the insurance company.

If all of this fails, remember that the patient or guarantor is responsible for any remaining charges. Bear in mind that if the rehabilitation facility accepts assignment of payment from a CMS fiscal intermediary, the facility is prohibited from collecting any payment from the patient.

REHABILITATION PATIENT DOCUMENTATION

Patient note documentation is more than adequately explained in other chapters of this text. There are aspects of patient notes that, if included, will make reimbursement easier. To be redundant, document all procedures and modalities used. Otherwise, to payers, the treatment didn't occur.

In the initial visit or initial evaluation note, write an appropriate history that can be referred to when setting goals. Record the results of the evaluation, including what was found as well as those signs and symptoms that were not seen but may have been expected, given the history. Perform and describe the results of a functional evaluation based on the patient or provider goals ("patient was unable to toe-raise on left foot and ankle"). List the body parts to be treated, modalities or procedures that may be used, and expected frequency and number of treatment sessions. Establish a prognosis and declare patient and provider goals, both short-term and long-term. Provider goals should be functional, measurable, and time-based. Finally, state whether there are any barriers to learning by the patient (language, disability, etc) and that the treatment plan was discussed and approved by the patient and/or guardian if the athlete is a minor.

Use daily treatment records to document modalities or procedures used and the patient's response to them. Write down any changes in patient status relevant to the diagnosis or prognosis. Reevaluate the patient every 30 days or if a significant intervening event occurs. The reevaluation note does not need to be as detailed as the initial evaluation note, but it must be based on the findings of the initial evaluation. Finally, it should include any changed goals or prescriptions. Copies of the initial evaluation notes and subsequent reevaluation notes should be sent to the physician's office for inclusion in his/her files.

SUMMARY

Documentation for reimbursement is a time-consuming and, ironically, a nonreimbursable activity. It is in the best interest of the athletic trainer responsible for reim-

---

Common Mistake #1

Documenting treatment interventions for patients whose medical condition falls outside the scope of practice for an athletic trainer

Suggestion for avoidance: Know the practice act for the state you work in so that you are legally treating all patients.

Common Mistake #2

Not updating patient information forms

Suggestion for avoidance: Patient information forms should be updated annually at minimum. Formally developing a process that requests any changes in patient/athlete information is a good idea.

Common Mistake #3

Not becoming familiar with standardized documentation forms for reimbursement

Suggestion for avoidance: Even though you may not work in a reimbursable setting, documentation standards are very similar. You should be aware of what the highest standards are as a general practice rule.

---

bursement to stay as knowledgeable as possible on coding, billing processes, reimbursement trends, and changes in CMS policies. Seminars, workshops, and in-services are offered on these topics. Even though athletic trainers are not recognized by CMS as approved providers, many health insurance payers follow the lead of CMS when it comes to making decisions about who gets reimbursed for doing what.

A quick check online for medical billing companies revealed over 127,000 entries. Outsourcing the billing process may be well worth the additional cost in lieu of time spent and frustration expended. A similar check for rehabilitation documentation software showed over 26,000 entries. Timesaving mechanisms exist that could ease the burden of documentation. For athletic trainers, it is gratifying to know that services once offered at no cost, other than to the employer, may now be paid for, in similar fashion to other allied health care professionals.

DISCUSSION ITEMS

Using the information presented in this chapter, answer the following:

1. What are the laws in your state regarding reimbursement for athletic training services? How does this effect your documentation style?

2. What is a third-party payer? What influence does a third-party payer have on the way you document your treatment interventions?

3. Does your institution use a patient encounter form of any style? Have you ever examined it carefully? If you currently have one, what suggestions do you have to improve this form?

4. Does your institution currently use a patient/athlete information form? How often is it updated?

5. What is the difference between a CPT code and an ICD-9 code? What is the relationship between documentation and these codes?

6. What suggestions do you have for improving your documentation styles to avoid denials of reimbursement?

7. The "8 minute rule" may be something totally unfamiliar to you in the university athletic training setting. If this became a standard issue for delivery of services to university athletes, what impact do you think it would have on health care?

Konin JG, Frederick MA. *Documentation for Athletic Training*. Thorofare, NJ: SLACK Incorporated; 2005.

National Athletic Trainers' Association Board of Certification Standards for Documentation

The following are minimal standards. Each one is essential for the practice of athletic training.

Standard 1: Direction

The athletic trainer renders service or treatment under the direction of a physician or dentist.

Standard 2: Injury and On-Going Care Services

All services should be documented in writing by the athletic trainer and shall become part of the athlete's permanent records.

Standard 3: Documentation

The athletic trainer shall accept responsibility for recording details of the athlete's health status. Documentation shall include:

1. Athlete's name and any other identifying information
2. Referral source (doctor, dentist)
3. Date, initial assessment, results, and database
4. Program plan and estimated length
5. Program methods, results, and revisions
6. Date of discontinuation and summary
7. Athletic trainer's signature

SYMBOLS AND MEDICAL TERMINOLOGY ABBREVIATIONS

SYMBOLS

↑	increase
↓	decrease
↔	to and from
1°	primary
2°	secondary, secondary to
@	at
+	plus, positive
-	minus
±	plus or minus
=	equals
>	greater than
<	less than
#	number
//	parallel or parallel bars
/	per
/d	per day
%	percent
∧	perpendicular
1x	one time
+, et.	and
+1	assistance (assistance of 1 person given)

A

a.	artery
ā	before
A, acc	accommodation
(A)	assisted, assistance
A:	Assessment
AAROM	active assistive range of motion
abd	abduction
Ab	antibody
AB, ab	abortion
ABC	aspiration biopsy cytology

ABGs	arteriole blood gases
ABLB	alternate binatural loudness balance
abnorm.	abnormal
ABR	absolute bed rest
ABR	auditory brainstem response
ac	before meals
AC	acromioclavicular
AC	air conduction
AC	anticoagulant
ACI	approved clinic instructor
AC jt.	acromioclavicular joints
ACL	anterior cruciate ligament
ACS	American Cancer Society
ACTH	adrenocorticotrophic hormone
AD	admitting diagnosis
AD	right ear
ADA	Americans with Disabilities Act
add.	adduction
ADD	attention deficit disorder
ADH	antidiuretic hormone
ADL	activities of daily living
ad lib	as desired
ad lib	at discretion
adm	admission
ADM	administration
AE	above elbow
AF	atrial fibrillation
AFO	ankle foot orthosis
Ag	antigen
AI	autistic impaired
AIDS	acquired immune deficiency syndrome
AIIS	anterior inferior iliac spine
AJ	ankle jerk
AK, A/K	above knee
A/K Amp	above-knee amputation
ALOS	average length of stay
Am, A.M.	morning
AMA	against medical advice

AMA	American Medical Association
amb	ambulation
am't	amount
ANS	autonomic nervous system
Ant	anterior
AODM	adult-onset diabetes mellitus
A&P	auscultation and percussion
AP	anterior-posterior
approx, ~	approximately
appts.	appointments
APTA	American Physical Therapy Association
ARDS	adult respiratory distress syndrome
ARF	acute renal failure
AROM	active range of motion
ART	active resistive training
As, Ast, astigm	astigmatism
AS	left ear (auris sinistra)
ASC	athletic trainer, certified
ASAP	as soon as possible
ASHD	arteriosclerotic heart disease
ASIS	anterior superior iliac spine
ASROM	assistive range of motion
Ath	athlete
ATNR	asymmetrical tonic neck reflex
AU	both ears
AV	atrioventricular; arteriovenous

B

B, (B), bil., bilat	bilateral
B, (B)	both
Ba	barium
BADL	basic activities of daily living
BaE	barium enema
BE	base equivalent
BE	below elbow
BG	blood glucose
Bid, b.i.d.	twice a day
BIN	twice at night
BK	below knee
BK Amp, BKA	below-knee amputation
Bl	blood
BLE	both lower extremities
bm	body mechanics
BM	bowel movement
BMD	bone mineral density
BMI	body mass index
BMR	basal metabolic rate
BP	blood pressure
bpm	beats per minute

BRP	bathroom privileges
BS	blood sugar
B/S	bedside
BSA	body surface area
BT	bleeding time
BT	brain tumor
BUE	both upper extremities
BUN	blood urea nitrogen test
Bx	biopsy

C

$\bar{c}$, w/	with
C	cervical
C°	Centigrade, Celsius
C1	first cervical vertebra
Ca	calcium
CA	cancer, carcenoma
CABG	coronary artery bypass graft
CAD	coronary artery disease
cal	calories
CARF	Commission on Accreditation of Rehabilitation Facilities
CAT	computer-assisted tomography
CAT scan	computed axial tomography scan
Cath	catheter
CBC	complete blood count
CBI	closed brain injury
CBR	complete bed rest
CBS	chronic brain syndrome
cc	cubic centimeters
CC, C/C	chief complaint
CCU	coronary care unit
CDC	Centers for Disease Control and Prevention
CE	continuing education
CEU	continuing education units
CF	cystic fibrosis
CHD	coronary heart disease
CHF	congestive heart failure
CHI	closed head injury
CHT	certified hand therapist
CI	cardiac index
CI	clinical instructor
Cl	chlorine
cm	centimeter
CMP	competitive medical plan
CNS	central nervous system
c/o	complains of
CO	carbon monoxide
CO_2	carbon dioxide
COG	center of gravity

COLD	chronic obstructive lung disease
COM	center of mass, center of motion
Cont., cont	continue
Contra	contraindication
COPD	chronic obstructive pulmonary disease
COTA	certified occupational therapy assistant
CP	cerebral palsy
CP	chest pain
CP	compression pump
CPE	continuing professional education
CPM	continuous passive motion
CPR	cardiopulmonary resuscitation
c.r.	contract-relax
CRI	chronic renal insufficiency
C&S	culture and sensitivity
CSF	cerebral spinal fluid
CT scan	computed tomography scan
CTS	carpal tunnel syndrome
cu	cubic
CV	cardiovascular
CVA	cerebrovascular accident
CVD	cardiovascular disease
CWI	crutch walking instructions
CXR	chest x-ray
Cysto	cystoscopic examination

D

dc	discontinue
d/c	discharged
DD	developmental disabilities
DDD	degenerative disc disease
dep	dependent
DEP	data, evaluation, performance goals
dept.	department
derm	dermatology
DI	diabetes insipidus
DI	diagnostic imaging
dia	diameter
diff	differential count (white blood cells)
DIP	distal interphalangeal joint
DJD	degenerative joint disease
dl	deciliter
DM	diabetes mellitus
DNKA	did not keep appointment
DNR	do not resuscitate order
DO	doctor of osteopathy
DOA	dead on arrival
DOB	date of birth
Doff	take off clothing
DOMS	delayed onset muscle soreness

Don	put on clothing
DPT	Doctor of Physical Therapy
Dr	doctor
dsg.	dressing
DTR	deep tendon reflex
DVT	deep venous thrombosis
DX	diagnosis
DZ	disease

E

EAP	employee assistance program
ECF	extended care facility
ECF, E.C.F	extracellular fluid
ECG, EKG	electrocardiogram
ECHO	echocardiogram
ECU	environmental control unit
EDM	extensor digitorum minimi
EEG	electroencephalogram
EENT	ear, eyes, nose, and throat
EMA	external moment arm
EMG	electromyogram
EMS	electrical muscle stimulation
EMS	emergency medical services
ENT	ear, nose, and throat
EOB	edge of bed
EOB	explanation of benefits
EOM	edge of mat
EOM	extraocular movement
EPL	extensor pollicis longus
ER, ext rot	external rotation
E.R., ER	emergency room
ERV	expiratory reserve volume
ES	electrical stimulation
EST	electric shock therapy
ESTR	electrical stimulation for tissue repair
etc	and so on
etiol	etiology
ETOH	alcohol
ev	eversion
eval	evaluation, evaluate
ex.	exercise
Ex	example
ext	extension

F

F, ♀	female
F	Fahrenheit
F	fair (muscle strength, balance)
FAROM	functional active range of motion

FAS	fetal alcohol syndrome
FBS	fasting blood sugar
FCU	flexor carpi ulnaris
FDA	Food and Drug Administration
FEF	forced expiratory flow
FEMS	functional electrical muscle stimulation
FES	functional electrical stimulation
FEV	forced expiratory volume
FH	family history
flex	flexion
FOR	frame of reference
FOR	functional outcome report
FRG	functional related groups
ft	foot, feet (the measurement, not the body part)
F/U	follow-up
Func	function
FUO	fever, unknown origin
FVC	forced vital capacity
FWB	full weight bearing
FWW, fw/w	front wheeled walker
Fx	fracture (d)
FY	fiscal year

G

G	good (muscle strength, balance)
G, gm	gram
GAS	general adaptation syndrome
gastroc	gastrocnemius muscles
GB	gallbladder
GC	gonorrhea
GCS	Glasgow Coma Scale
GER	gerontology
GH	glenohumeral
GI	gastrointestinal
gluts	gluteals
GMT	gross muscle test
Gr.	grain
GSH, GSW	gun shot wound
Gt.	gait
gtt	drops
GU	genitourinary
GYN	gynecology

H

h, hr., hr	hour
H2	histamine
HA, H/A	headache
HAb	horizontal abduction

HAd	horizontal adduction
hams	hamstrings
HAV	Hepatitis A virus
Hb, Hgb, HGB	hemoglobin
HBP	high blood pressure
HBV	Hepatitis B virus
HCT, hct, Ht	hematocrit
HCVD	hypertensive cardiovascular disease
HDL	high-density lipoprotein
HEA	Higher Education Act
HEENT	head, ear, eyes, nose, throat
hemi	hemiplegia
HF	heart failure
HEP	home exercise program
H&H, H/H	hematocrit and hemoglobin
HI	head injury
HI	hearing impaired
HIV	human immunodeficiency virus
HMO	health maintenance organization
HNP	herniated nucleus pulposus
H/O	history of
HOB	head of bead
horiz.	horizontal
H.P.	hot pack
H&P	history and physical
HPI	history of present illness
HR	heart rate
hs	at bedtime
HS	high school
HS	hours of sleep
HSV	herpes simplex virus
ht.	Height
HT	hubbard tank
Htn, HTN	hypertension
Hx, hx	history
Hypo	hypodermic
Hz	hertz

I

I	independently
I, indep	independent
IADL	instrumental activities of daily living
IBS	irritable bowel syndrome
IC	inspiratory capacity
ICF	intermediate care facility
ICF, I.C.F	intracellular fluid
ICP	intermittent compression pump
ICP	intracranial pressure
ICT	intermittent cervical traction
ICU	intensive care unit
ID	intradermal
I&D	incision and drainage

IDDM	insulin-dependent diabetes mellitus
IEP	individual education program
IH	infectious hepatitis
ILC	independent living center
IM	intramuscular
imp.	impression
in.	inches
ind.	indications
inf	inferior
inhal	inhalation
inj	injection
int.	internal
inv	inversion
I&O	intake and output
IP	interphalangeal
IPTX	intermittent pelvic traction
IQ	intelligence quotient
IR	internal rotation
IRV	inspiratory reserve volume
IS	intercostal space
IU	international unit(s)
IV	intravenous
IVF	inferior vena cava

J

JCAHO	Joint Commission on Accreditation of Healthcare Organizations
JOMACI	judgment, orientation, memory, abstraction, and calculation
JRA	junior rheumatoid arthritis
JROM	joint range of motion
Jt	joint
JW	jumpwalker

K

KAFO	knee, ankle, foot orthosis
KB	kilobyte
kcal	kilocalories
kg	kilogram
KJ	knee jerk
KO	knee orthosis
KUB	kidney, ureter, and bladder

L

L, lt.	left
L, l.	liter
L1	first lumbar vertebra
L5	Fifth lumbar vertebra

L&A	light and accommodation
LA	left atrium
lat.	lateral
lat. bar	latissimus dorsi bar
lb., #	pound
LBP	low back pain
LCL	lateral collateral ligament
LD	learning disabilities
LDL	low-density lipoprotein
LE	lower extremity
lg	large
LLB	long leg brace
LLC	long leg cast
LLD	leg length discrepancy
LLE	left lower extremity
LLQ	left lower quadrant
LMNL	lower motor neuron lesion
LMP	last menstrual period
LOA	leave of absence
LOB	loss of balance
LOC	loss of consciousness
LOS	length of stay
LP	lumbar puncture
LPN	licensed practical nurse
LRQ	lower right quadrant
LS	lumbosacral
LTC	long-term care
LTG	long-term goals
LUE	left upper extremity
LUL	left upper lobe
LV	left ventricle
L&W	living and well

M

M, ♂	male
m	meter
m, mm	muscle
ma	milliampere
MA	mechanical advantage
MAS	mobile arm support
max	maximum
MBD	minimal brain damage
MC	metacarpal
MCA	motorcycle accident
MCE	medical care evaluation
mcg	micrograms
MCL	medial collateral ligament
MCO	managed care organization
MD	medical doctor; doctor of medicine
M.D.	muscular dystrophy
med	medial
med	median
med	medium

MED	minimal effective dose
MED	minimal erythemal dose
Meds.	medications
MFR	myofascial release
MFT	muscle function test
mg	milligram
MH	mental health
MH	moist heat
MI	myocardial infarction
MICU	medical intensive care unit
min	minimal
min	minimum
min.	minute
ml, mL	milliliters
mm	millimeter
mmHG	millimeters of mercury
MMT	manual muscle test
mo.	month
mod	moderate
MP, MCP	metacarpal-phalangeal, metacarpal-phalangeal
mph	miles per hour
MRE	manual resistive exercise
MRI	magnetic resonance imaging
MS	multiple sclerosis
MS	mitral stenosis
MSP	Medicare secondary payer
MSQ	Mental status questionnaire
MTP	metatarsophalangeal
MUP	motor unit potential
MVA	motor vehicle accident
MVC	maximum voluntary contraction
MVE	maximum voluntary effort
MVP	mitral valve prolapse
Myop	myopia

N

n.	nerve
N	normal (muscle strength)
Na	sodium
N/A	not applicable
NDT	neural developmental treatment
neg., -	negative
neurosurg.	neurosurgery
N.H.	nursing home
NICU	neonatal intensive care unit
NIDDM	non-insulin-dependent diabetes mellitus
NKA	no known allergies
NKDA	no known drug allergies
noc.	night, by night

NPO	nothing by mount
NREM	non-rapid eye movement
NSAID	nonsteroidal anti-inflammatory drug
Nsg	nursing
NSR	normal sinus rhythm
NWB	nonweight bearing

O

O	none
O:	objective
O^2	oxygen
O x 3	oriented to person, place, and time
OA	osteoarthritis
OB	obstetrics
obs	observation
OBS	organic brain syndrome
OCS	orthopedic certified specialist
OD	right eye (oculus dexter)
OOB	out of bed
o.p.	overpressure
O.P., OP	outpatient
OPD	outpatient department
O.R.	operating room
ORIF	open reduction, internal fixation
ortho	orthopedics
os	mouth
OS	left eye (oculus sinister)
OT	occupational therapy, occupational therapists
OTC	over the counter
OTR	occupational therapist, registered
OTS	occupational therapist, student
OU	both eyes (oculus unitas)
oz.	ounce

P

p̄	after
p	post
P	poor (muscle strength, balance)
P:	plan (treatment plan)
P+	pain
P-	pain absent
PA, P-A	posterior/anterior
P.A.	physician's assistant
PAMs	physical agent modalities
para	paraplegia
path	pathology
p̄c, pp	after meals

PCA	personal care attendant	PTB cast	patellar tendon bearing cast
PCL	posterior cruciate ligament	PTB prosth	patellar tendon bearing prosthesis
P/D flex	plantarflexion/ dorsiflexion	PTSD	post-traumatic stress disorder
PD	physical disabilities	PUW	pick up walker
PDD	persuasive developmental disorder	PVD	peripheral vascular disease
PDR	*Physician Desk Reference*	PWA	person with AIDS
Pe, Px	physical examination	PWB	partial weight bearing
PE	pulmonary embolism		
peds	pediatrics		
per	by		
per	through		

Q

per os, p.o	by mouth
PERRL	pupils, equal, round, reactive to light
PET	positron emission testing
PFT	Pulmonary function testing and accommodations

q	every
QA	quality assurance
qd	every day
QEE	quadriceps extension exercises
qh	every hour
QI	quality improvement
Qid, 4xd	four times a day
qn	every night
qns	quantity not significant
qod	every other day
qt.	quart
quad	quadriplegia
quads	quadriceps

P.H.	past history
Phys	physical, physiology
PI	present illness
PICU	pediatric intensive care unit
PID	pelvic inflammatory disease
PIIS	posterior inferior iliac spine
PIP	proximal interphalangeal joint
PM, p.m.	afternoon
PMH	past medical history
PMR	physical medicine and rehabilitation
PNI	peripheral nerve injury
PNF	proprioceptive neuromuscular facilitation

R

Rt	right
RA	reasonable accommodations
RA	rheumatoid arthritis
RAM	rapid alternating movements
RBC	red blood cell count
RC	rehabilitation counselor
RCL	radial collateral ligament
R.D.	registered dietician
RD	respiratory disease
RDL	romanian deadlift
RDS	respiratory distress syndrome
re:	regarding
rehab	rehabilitation
REM	rapid eye movement
reps	repetitions
resp	respiratory, respiration
ret.	return
RET	rational emotive therapy
RF	rheumatoid factor
RHD	rheumatic heart disease
RLE	right lower extremity
RLL	right lower lobe
RLQ	right lower quadrant
RM	repeated movements
RM	repetition maximum

PNS	Peripheral nervous system
PO	postoperative
POMR	problem-oriented medical record
pos.	positive
poss.	possible
post-op	after surgery (operation)
PPE	personal protective equipment
PPO	preferred provider organization
PRE	progressive resistive exercise
pre-op, preop	before surgery (operation)
prn	whenever necessary
PRO	peer review organization
Prog	prognosis
PROM	passive range of motion
prox	proximal
PSIS	posterior superior iliac spine
PSP	problem, status, plan
PSPG	problem, status, plan, goals
Psych	psychiatry
pt	pint
Pt., pt	patient
PT	physical therapy, physical therapists
PTA	physical therapist assistant
PTA	prior to admission
PTB	patellar tendon bearing

RN	registered nurse	Sm	symptoms
R.O., r/o	rule out	SMI	supplemental medical insurance
ROM	range of motion	SNF	skilled nursing facility
ROS	review of systems	SNS	somatic nervous system
rot. x	rotation	SOAP	subjective, objective, assessment, and plan
RPE	rate of perceived exertion		
RPT	registered physical therapist	SOB	shortness of breath
RPTA	registered physical therapist assistant	soln	solution
RROM	resistive range of motion	SOMR	source-oriented medical record
R.T.	respiratory therapist	SOP	standard operating procedure
RTI	routine task inventory	sos	if necessary
RUE	right upper extremity	sp gr, SG	specific gravity
RUQ	right upper quadrant	Sp	speech
RV	residual volume	S.P., S/P	status post
Rx	prescription	spec	specimen
Rx	therapy	SPEM	smooth pursuit eye movement
		SPSS	Statistical Package for Social Sciences
		SPT	student physical therapist
		SPTx	static pelvic traction

S

s, w/o	without	sq	square
S	supervision	sqt	squat
S1	first sacral vertebra	SSI	supplemental security income
SAC	short arm cast	S.T.	speech therapy
SACH	solid ankle cushion heel	stat.	immediately, at once
SAD	seasonal affective disorder	STD	sexually transmitted disease
SAQ	short arc quad	STG	short-term goal
Sat	saturated	STNR	symmetrical tonic neck reflex
SBA	standby assist	str.	strength
subcu, subq	subcutaneous	strep	streptooccus
s.c.	subcutaneously	STSG	split thickness skin graft
S̄C	sternoclavicular	sup	superior
SCI	spinal cord injury	surg	surgery
SC joint	sternoclavicular joint	SWD	shortwave diathermy
SCS	sports certified specialist	Sup	supination
SCTx	static cervical traction	Sx	signs
SE	side effects		
sec.	seconds		
SEC	single-end cane		
SED	seriously emotionally disturbed		
SED	suberythemal dose		
sh	shoulder		

T

SI	sacroiliac	T, temp.	temperature
SI	sensory integration	T	trace (muscle strength)
SICU	surgical intensive care unit	T1	first thoracic vertebra
SIDS	sudden infant death syndrome	T&A	tonsils and adenoids
sig	directions for use	TAB	temporarily abled body
sig	give as follows	tab	tablet
SLB	short leg brace	TAP	turning and positioning program
sld. bd.	sliding board	TB	tuberculosis
SLP	speech language pathologist	TBI	traumatic brain injury
SLR	straight leg raise	TBSA	total body surface area
SLWC	short leg walking cast	tbsp.	tablespoon
		TDD	telecommunication device for the deaf
		TDD	tentative discharge date

TDP	tentative discharge plan
TDWB	touch down weight bearing
TFCC	triangular fibrocartilage complex
THA	total hip arthroplasty
TENS, TNS	transcutaneous electrical nerve stimulator
ther. ex.	therapeutic exercise
THR	total hip replacement
TIA	transient ischemic attack
tid	three times a day
TJM	temporomandibular joint
TKA	total knee arthroplasty
TKE	terminal knee extension
TKR	total knee replacement
TLSO	thoracic lumbar sacral orthosis
TNR	tonic neck reflex
t.o.	telephone order
TOWER	testing, orientation, and work evaluation in rehabilitation
TPR	temperature, pulse, and respiration
TQM	total quality management
trng.	training
tsp.	teaspoon
TSS	toxic shock syndrome
TT	tilt table
TTWB	toe touch weight bearing
TTY	teletypewriter
TUR	transurethral resection
TV	tidal volume
TWB	touch weight bearing
Tx, Rx	treatment

U

U	units
UA	urine analysis
UCL	ulnar collateral ligament
UE	upper extremity
UED1	upper extremity diagonal 1
UGI	upper gastrointestinal
U&L, U/L	upper and lower
ULQ	upper left quadrant
UMN	upper motor neuron
UMNL	upper motor neuron lesion
Un	unable
ung	ointment
URI	upper respiratory infection
URQ	upper right quadrant
US	ultrasound
UTI	urinary tract infection
UV	ultraviolet

V

VA	visual acuity
VC	visual capacity
V.D.	venereal disease
VER	visual evoked response
vert.	vertical
VF	visual field
VI	volume index
VLDL	very-low-density liopoproteins
v.o., VO	verbal orders
vol.	volume
v.s., vs	vital signs

W

WBC	white blood cell count
WBQC	wide-based quad cane
w/c, WC	wheelchair
W/cm^2	watts per square centimeter
WFL	within functional limits
WHO	wrist hand orthosis
WNL	within normal limits
WP	whirlpool
w/u	work up

X

x	times, number of times performed
XX	female sex chromosomes
XY	male sex chromosomes

Y

yd.	yard
y/o, YO, y.o.	years old
yr.	year

PREFIXES/ SUFFIXES

a- (an-)	without
arthr-	joint (arthritis)
auto-	self
bi-	two; double (biceps)
brachi-, brachium-	arm
brevis-	short
capit-	head
cervix	neck

chrondro-	cartilage	BSW	A social worker
circum-	around	Cardiology	The study of the heart and its conditions
contra-	against; opposed		
costa-	rib	COT	Occupational Therapists
crux-	cross	COTA	Occupational Therapy Assistant
delta-	triangle		
di-	double, two	C.S.C.S	Certified Strength and Conditioning Specialist
dia-	through, completely		
dis-	seperation	Dermatology	The study of the skin
ect-	outside	D.C.	Doctor of Chiropractic (chiropractor)
-ectomy	excision, removal		
end-, ent-	within	DDS	Dentist
epi-	upon	DMD	Dentist
extra-	beyond, outward	D.O.	Doctor of Osteopathy
gastr-	stomach	D.P.M.	Doctor of Podiatric Medicine (Podiatrist)
hist-, histo-	tissue		
hydro-	water	E.M.T.	Emergency Medical Technician
hyper-	above; over		
hypo-	under; less	E.M.T.—P	Emergency Medical Technician—Paramedic
infra-	below		
intr-, intra	within	Etiology	The study of causes of injury and disease
medi-	middle		
meta-	changed, beyond	Exercise Physiologists	A scientist that works with the processes of physiological responses to exercise
micro-	small		
myo-	muscle		
nephr-	kidney	Gastroenterology	The study of the digestive tract
para-	beside	Gynecology	The study of female reproductive conditions
-physis	to grow		
post-	after, behind	L.M.T	Licensed massage therapist
pre-, pro-	before, in front of	L.P.N	Licensed Practical Nurse
re-	again, back	L.P.T.	Licensed Physical Therapist
rect-	straight	L.V.N	Licensed Vocational Nurse
ren-	kidney	M.A.	Medical Assistant/Master of Arts Degree
retro-	back, backward		
sect-	to cut	M.D.	Medical Doctor
sub-	under	M.Ed	Master of Education degree
super-	over, excessive	M.S.	Master of Science degree
supra-	above	MSW	Master of Social Work
sym-, syn-	together	Nephrology	The study of kidney conditions
teres	round, rope like	Neurology	The study of nervous system disorders
trans-	across, through		
ultra-	beyond, excess	Obstetrics	The study of pregnancy conditions
vert-, ventr-	belly, anterior		
		O.D.	Doctor of Optometry
		Oncology	The study of cancerous conditions

MEDICAL SPECIALTIES

A.T.C	Athletic Trainer, Certified	Opthalmologist	A medical doctor who deals with conditions of the eye, surgery
Anesthesiology	The study of anesthesia and the effects upon the body		
		Ophthalmology	The study of eye conditions
Biomechanist	A person with expertise in analysis of human movement	Optomistrist	A doctor who fits eyeglasses, contact lenses and prescribes medications

Orthopedics	The study of joint, bone and muscle conditions	P.T.A.	Physical Therapist Assistant
P.A.	Physician's Assistant	Proctology	The study of anal conditions
P.A.C.	A Certified Physician Assistant	Psychiatry	The study of mental conditions
Pathology	The study of the nature and cause of disease	Radiology	The practice that uses x-rays, MRI, etc
Pediatrics	The study of children's conditions	R.D.	Registered Dietician
Pharmacist	A person that selects, dispenses, gives dosage, and consults with the patient about side effects of medication	Respiratory Therapist	A person that works with patients to overcome and manage respiratory problems
		Rheumatology	The study of arthritic/joint conditions
Physiatrist	A person that specializes in physical rehabilitation/medicine	R.N.	Registered Nurse
		Sports Psychologist	A person that deals with the psychological issues that arise in athletes
Podiatrist	A person that specializes in foot and ankle conditions	Speech Therapist	A person that works with patients to overcome and manage speech/vocal problems
P.T.	Physical Therapist		

Observation

1. Deformity noted over the medial epicondyle of the athlete's right elbow.

2. Ecchymosis present over the left infraorbital rim secondary to being hit with a baseball.

3. Patient walks into the athletic training room cradling her left arm to her side, with deformity at the glenohumeral joint indicating a possible shoulder dislocation.

4. Athlete enters the facility nonweight bearing on his right leg, his knee locked into 45 degrees of flexion; his teammate was assisting him into the facility.

5. Throughout the history, the athlete seemed apprehensive and was shifting weight from foot to foot.

6. The athlete fell after being hit by another football player; he presented with deformity to his right forearm.

7. The athlete presents with scapular winging on the left side.

8. The athlete returned from the doctor with a diagnosis of kyphosis.

9. The patient reported to the athletic training room 2 weeks post-ACL reconstruction surgery and had significant muscle wasting to her affected quadriceps muscle.

10. The patient had a cyanotic coloring to the skin on her face after experiencing a fainting episode.

11. The wrestler came into the athletic training room with his left eye dropped in its eye socket, secondary to a zygomatic fracture.

12. The soccer player exhibited exostosis on his left calcaneus.

13. The basketball player came into the facility cradling his arm at 60 degrees of flexion.

Konin JG, Frederick MA. *Documentation for Athletic Training*. Thorofare, NJ: SLACK Incorporated; 2005.

Palpation

1. The athlete exhibited point tenderness over the medial epicondyle of his right elbow.

2. The athlete complained of pain when the lateral joint line of her right knee was palpated.

3. Movement and crepitus were felt over the 5th metacarpal. The athlete said that he punched a wall, leading to a possible boxer's fracture.

4. The patient complained of increased tenderness when the spinous process of the 5th lumbar vertebrae was compressed.

5. The athlete experienced discomfort during palpation of the lateral collateral ligament of her knee.

6. Point tenderness over the prominent medial tubercle of the calcaneus, indicating a possible bone spur in this location.

7. The athlete complained of increased pain when the anatomical snuffbox was palpated.

8. The patient experienced point tenderness over the acromioclavicular joint of her right shoulder.

9. There is crepitus and pain during palpation of the fifth through ninth ribs on the left side.

10. Pain and inflammation over the anterior talofibular ligament of his left ankle secondary to an inversion ankle sprain.

Konin JG, Frederick MA. *Documentation for Athletic Training*. Thorofare, NJ: SLACK Incorporated; 2005.

Head/Face

1. Patient presented with hyphema in the anterior chamber of the eye, referral indicated.

2. The athlete came to the athletic training room after the football game complaining of a headache. Upon examination, an area of discoloration over the mastoid area called Battle's sign was noticed.

3. When we arrived on the scene, the athlete was exhibiting decorticate posturing, with the arms, wrists, and fingers flexed, and adducted, and the legs extended, medially rotated, and plantar flexed.

4. The athlete could not maintain a contraction when asked to bite on a tongue depressor, which is indicative of a mandibular fracture.

5. An orange halo appeared around the blood on the gauze pad while attending the downed athlete, which indicates cerebrospinal fluid mixed with blood.

6. During the cranial examination, it was found that the patient had adequate near acuity, but could not make out the score on the scoreboard.

7. The athlete presented with a depressed left eye with limitation of upward and downward movements, secondary to a blow out fracture of the left orbital floor.

8. The collegiate wrestler exhibits hematoma auris, a keloid scar in the auricle due to friction or twisting of the ear.

9. The athlete comes to the athletic training room with a foreign object in his eye, which was removed by inverting the eyelid.

10. The athlete presents with a maxillary fracture, with anteroposterior rocking of the upper teeth.

Konin JG, Frederick MA. *Documentation for Athletic Training*. Thorofare, NJ: SLACK Incorporated; 2005.

Neck

1. While performing the vertebral artery test, patient became dizzy and slurred her speech, indicating a partial or complete occlusion of the vertebral artery.

2. During a neurological exam after trauma, the athlete was found to have parathesia along the C7 dermatome.

3. Normal cervical spine active range of motion in extension, rotation, and lateral flexion; however, flexion is restricted to 15 degrees.

4. During resistive range of motion, all directions were 5 out of 5, with the exception of resisted lateral flexion to the left, which was 3 out of 5.

5. A diminished C5 reflex was found in the right arm during the on-the-field examination of the athlete, which led to the decision to stabilize and transport to the hospital.

6. The athlete came into the facility complaining of sharp pain along the right arm, which was relieved when placed on intermittent mechanical traction.

7. During the on-the-field examination, point tenderness was detected over the C6 spinous process.

8. When the athlete was told to swallow, she reported dysphagia, which could be indicative of an anterior vertebral subluxation.

9. During the cervical spine evaluation, the foraminal compression test was administered, with an increase in the pain level on the same side as the head was laterally flexed.

10. Patient was put on traction to ease neck discomfort, but could not stand the pressure on his recently dislocated temporomandibular joint.

Konin JG, Frederick MA. *Documentation for Athletic Training*. Thorofare, NJ: SLACK Incorporated; 2005.

Shoulder

1. Athlete was not able to complete the drop arm test, his arm fell to his side and the athlete complained of pain.

2. The Hawkins-Kennedy test for impingement elicited pain when performed on the swimmer, who was suspected of having a bicipital impingement.

3. During palpation of the clavicle, the athlete complained of pain. The piano key sign was then administered and found to be positive.

4. During the shoulder evaluation, the patient exhibited a positive anterior apprehension test, but showed less discomfort during the Jobe relocation test, which suggests an anterior shoulder dislocation.

5. The quarterback was injured on the play, and when examined on the sideline, was found to have a positive O'Brien test, which lead to a probable diagnosis of a left labral tear.

6. The athlete could not complete the Roos test, and therefore may be suffering from thoracic outlet syndrome.

7. The cheerleader came into the athletic training room cradling her left arm against her body with her right arm, a protective posture.

8. The athlete exhibited a step deformity to his left shoulder after the anterior dislocation and subsequent capsular damage.

9. During active range of motion, the athlete complained of pain in an arc of abduction, from approximately 60 to 120 degrees, which could indicate tendonitis of the rotator cuff muscles.

10. The gymnast came into the athletic training room with a deformity of his biceps muscle secondary to a long head biceps disruption.

11. The athlete reported to the facility with his shoulder internally rotated and adducted, in the position of Erb's palsy.

12. The athlete complained of point tenderness during palpation of the acromioclavicular joint.

Konin JG, Frederick MA. *Documentation for Athletic Training*. Thorofare, NJ: SLACK Incorporated; 2005.

Lumbar/S1 Joint

1. The athlete came into the athletic training room with a shortened stride on the left side due to pain of the lumbar spine.

2. The patient presents with a forward flexed posture, laterally flexed to the left, away from the painful area on the right lower back.

3. The athlete presented with Faun's beard; a sign of spina bifida occulta.

4. The athlete exhibited painful and limited active extension of the lumbar spine.

5. During the examination, the left hip dropped while standing on the right leg, exhibiting a positive Trendelenburg sign.

6. The athlete has an equal apparent leg length, but in the functional leg length test, the left leg was ¼ inch longer than the right leg.

7. The athlete complained of pain during the straight leg-raising test at 50 degrees, increased with ankle dorsiflexion, indicates possible nerve root or sciatic nerve involvement.

8. The athlete is point tender over the left posterior superior iliac spine, which is also hypomobile during hip flexion.

9. When asked to perform the valsalva maneuver, the athlete complained of increased pain in the lumbar spine.

10. The athlete showed no pressure on the opposite heel when attempting a straight leg raise, which could be indicalative of malingering.

Konin JG, Frederick MA. *Documentation for Athletic Training*. Thorofare, NJ: SLACK Incorporated; 2005.

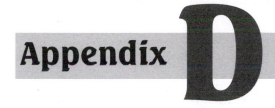
WORKSHEETS FOR DOCUMENTATION WRITING STYLES

Instructions: For each of the following sentences, rewrite the sentence in an abbreviated form using the correct medical terminology and symbols.

History

1. The athlete is a 24-year-old male, with no past medical history of stomach disorders.

2. The athlete complains of a sharp pain in the right lower quadrant of the abdomen.

3. The athlete states that pain increases with repeated movement of the right leg.

4. The athlete complains of shortness of breath after moderate cardiovascular training of approximately 20 minutes at 70 percent maximum heart rate.

5. The patient states that pain is decreased from 8 out of 10 to 2 out of 10 with static cervical traction.

6. The patient stated that his pain increased from 5 out of 10 to 9 out of 10 with ambulation on his right ankle.

7. The patient has a past medical history of anterior cruciate ligament deficiency and correction in the left leg.

8. Patient complains of diplopia, or double vision, secondary to a Le Fort I fracture.

Konin JG, Frederick MA. *Documentation for Athletic Training*. Thorofare, NJ: SLACK Incorporated; 2005.

9. The athlete states that he felt a crack when his ankle inverted and dorsiflexed.

10. The athlete's chief complaint is loss of range of motion in the right knee, combined with a locking of the right knee when full extension is attempted.

11. The athlete came to the athletic training room after hitting her head on the basketball court.

12. The athlete complains of low back pain beginning after being hit from behind during football practice.

13. The athlete came to the athletic trainer complaining of burning pain beginning in his left shoulder and radiating to his fingers.

14. The athlete came out of practice complaining of sudden photophobia and nausea.

15. The athlete complains of his right knee giving away when going down stairs.

16. The athlete complained of numbness in his fingers after typing a paper for class.

17. The athlete discontinued practice complaining of pain in bilateral shins after increasing mileage from 5 to 7 miles daily.

18. Athlete's parents called and are concerned because the athlete has lost 20 pounds, while increasing her workouts to 3 times each day.

19. The patient complained of chronic left ankle instability.

Hip

1. The athlete complained of increased pain during the FABER test, which could indicate hip joint pathology.

2. The athlete complained of pain at the lateral femoral condyle at 30 degrees of knee flexion during Renne's test, indicating a possible irritation of the iliotibial band.

3. Tomorrow the athlete will report to the athletic training room to repeat the Thomas test, which was positive post-game for hip contractures.

4. The athlete complained of tenderness in the belly of the hamstrings group, as well as point tenderness isolated in the semitendinosis muscle.

5. We are treating the thigh contusion conservatively with ice, rest, and padding to try and avoid myositis ossificans.

6. The athlete has point tenderness and swelling over the lateral aspect of the greater trochanter secondary to trochanteric bursitis.

7. The young athlete was diagnosed with Legg-Calve-Perthes disease, an avascular necrosis of the femoral head, and was placed on bedrest.

8. The volleyball athlete was fitted with an orthoplast pad over her iliac crest after receiving a hip pointer during the game.

9. When observing the athlete laterally, it was noticed that the pelvis is anteriorly tilted due to increased lumbar lordosis.

Konin JG, Frederick MA. *Documentation for Athletic Training.* Thorofare, NJ: SLACK Incorporated; 2005.

Knee

1. The athlete underwent magnetic resonance imaging, and the doctor diagnosed her with the "unhappy triad" or a torn medial meniscus, medial collateral ligament, and anterior cruciate ligament.

2. The athlete received a four out of five when testing knee extension, showing weakness of the quadriceps group.

3. The athlete could not reach full knee extension because the tibia was not externally rotating to allow the screw home mechanism to take place.

4. The athlete could not support weight on his left knee, and was carried into the athletic training facility by 2 of his teammates.

5. The athlete complained of point tenderness during palpation of gerdy's tubercle.

6. The athlete had minimal opening of the joint during the varus stress test at 0 degrees, but the joint opening was significant when the knee was moved to 30 degrees of flexion, indicating lateral collateral ligament involvement.

7. During the on-the-field evaluation of the athlete's knee, the lachman's test was positive for an anterior cruciate ligament tear. This test was falsely negative after the game in the athletic training room due to hamstring guarding.

8. During measurement for the knee brace after the anterior cruciate ligament surgery, the athlete was found to have 3 centimeters of atrophy at 2 centimeters above the joint line, and 8 centimeters of atrophy at 10 centimeters above the joint line. The gastrocnemius muscles remained balanced.

9. The athlete was found to have an increased Q angle of 30 degrees, which could predispose her to poor patellar tracking.

10. The athlete fell to the ground, and the athletic trainer saw that her patella had dislocated laterally. She was splinted and referred to the hospital.

Konin JG, Frederick MA. *Documentation for Athletic Training.* Thorofare, NJ: SLACK Incorporated; 2005.

22. Athlete got injured in the intersquad game during the evening practice. He stated, "When I tried to tackle and stretched my leg out, I felt a sharp pain in my right groin." He is a defender. He walked out from the field by himself with limping. He has no history of groin injury. He did not hear any unusual sounds.

23. Athlete's skin temperature is within normal limits, neurological exam intact. Athlete's active range of motion is within normal limits with pain in plantarflexion/inversion. Passive range of motion has the same results, resistive range of motion is full with pain in plantarflexion, inversion, and eversion. Manual muscle testing reveals true deficits of 3 out of 5. Athlete complains of point tenderness over anterior talofibular ligament. Anterior drawer test positive for pain only. Talar tilt test positive for both pain and laxity. Negative heel strike test. Negative apply compression test.

24. Activity modification, progress to full weight bearing as symptoms subside. Donut pad given, follow up with Dr. Smith as needed. Treatment: cold whirlpool, Achilles stretch, great toe stretch. No practice.

Konin JG, Frederick MA. *Documentation for Athletic Training.* Thorofare, NJ: SLACK Incorporated; 2005.

25. Treatment is as follows: warm whirlpool for 15 minutes, Achilles stretch 3 times for 30 seconds, towel range of motion in dorsiflexion, inversion, and eversion. Toe crunches 100 times. BAPS board level two 25 times clockwise and counter clockwise. Yellow theraband: 3 sets of 10 in plantar flexion, dorsiflexion, inversion, and eversion. One leg balance for 30 seconds 3 times. Cold whirlpool for 15 minutes.

26. Treatment is as follows: stationary bike for 15 minutes, static quadriceps contraction 30 times, static hamstring contraction 30 times. Straight leg raises with 5 pound cuff weight 3 sets of 10 repetitions in flexion, extension, abduction, and adduction. Physioball squats 3 sets of 10 repetitions. Lateral step downs off 4 inch step 3 sets of 10 repetitions. Terminal knee extensions with grey theratubing: 3 sets of 10 repetitions. Interferential stimulation with 100 percent scan with an ice pack for 20 minutes.

27. Athlete came into the training room complaining of pain in the anterior aspect of his left shoulder. Athlete stated unremarkable and gradual onset over past 3 days. Athlete complains of pain in anterior left shoulder with playing basketball and activities of daily living after playing. Athlete rates the pain as "dull at first, then sharp," 7 on a 1 to 10 scale. Athlete has a history of tendonitis in his left shoulder.

28. Athlete came into training room complaining of left knee pain that began a week ago. She notices the pain on both sides of her patella. It is worse when she does "explosive" movements and upon impact.

29. Athlete came into training room complaining of right quadriceps pain. She is tender to palpate in the upper quad/hip flexor area. She has pain when walking, running, and going up stairs. Athlete says most pain is when she is taking off on sprints or running during practice or games. She has a previous history of quadricep injuries the past 2 seasons.

Konin JG, Frederick MA. *Documentation for Athletic Training.* Thorofare, NJ: SLACK Incorporated; 2005.

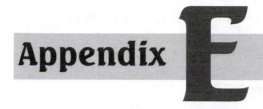

Appendix E

COMMONLY USED FORMS— INFORMATION FORMS

These forms consist of documents used to take biographical information mainly for contact purposes, health and family history, exit health information, and emergency contact information.

CONTENTS

JAMES MADISON UNIVERSITY INTERCOLLEGIATE ATHLETICS

DEPARTMENT OF SPORTS MEDICINE

ATHLETE INFORMATION FORM
2003-2004

Personal Information:

_____

Last Name   First Name   Middle Initial   Preferred Name

_____   _____
Social Security Number/Student ID Number   Sport

_____   Gender: Male   Female
Date of Birth

_____   _____
Campus Address   Campus Phone

_____   _____
Campus Email   Cell Phone

Permanent Home Address:

_____
Street Address

_____   _____
City   State   Zip Code   Country

_____   _____
Home Phone   Home Email

Emergency Contact Information:

_____   _____
First Name   Last Name   First Name   Last Name

_____   _____
Home Phone Number   Home Phone Number

_____   _____
Work Phone Number   Work Phone Number

_____   _____
Cell Phone Number   Cell Phone Number

_____   _____
Relation to Student Athlete   Relation to Student Athlete

Konin JG, Frederick MA. *Documentation for Athletic Training*. Thorofare, NJ: SLACK Incorporated; 2005.

James Madison University Intercollegiate Athletics
Department of Sports Medicine
Athletic Training Student Information Form
2004-2005

Personal Information:

Last Name	First Name	Middle Initial	Preferred Name

Social Security Number

Student ID Number

Date of Birth

Campus Email

Campus P. O. Box/Local Address

Campus or Local Phone Number

Cell Phone Number

Permanent Home Address:

Street Address	Town	State	Country

Home Telephone Number

Home\Parent(s) E-mail Address

Emergency Contact Information:

Last Name	First Name	Last Name	First Name

Home Phone\Cell Number

Home Phone\Cell Number

Work Phone Number

Work Phone Number

Relation

Relation

Address

Address

Konin JG, Frederick MA. *Documentation for Athletic Training*. Thorofare, NJ: SLACK Incorporated; 2005.

PRE-PARTICIPATION VETERAN SCREENING CONFIRMATION

NAME ______________________________ SS# _____________ DATE __________

ADDRESS ____

_________________________________ __________

TELEPHONE # ______________________________________

Please return this form as a confirmation of your participation. This form should be competed along with the BLUE packet, Health Information Update. The BLUE packet is extremely important and must be completed in it's entirety. Note that your parents signatures are required in several areas, along with other pertinent information. Please include a copy of your insurance card, front and back, with your insurance information.

If we do not receive this confirmation form, we will assume that you are not participating. In order for you to participate you must return all forms and have a screening performed by the athletic training staff at Salisbury State University. Your cooperation is very much appreciated.

TIME

DATE

A specific time will be given to you, in advance, once we receive this form .

Copyright © 2005 SLACK Incorporated. All rights reserved.
Konin JG, Frederick MA. *Documentation for Athletic Training.* Thorofare, NJ: SLACK Incorporated; 2005.

PRE-PARTICIPATION PHYSICAL EXAMINATION CONFIRMATION

NAME _____SS#_____ DATE_____

ADDRESS_____

_____

TELEPHONE # _____

Returning this form reserves a time for you to receive a **pre-participation physical examination** performed by SSU Medical Staff. Your coach will inform you of your specific time.

Complete all the information in the yellow packet, with the exception of the physical exam form. Please be prepared to pay $25.00 (check, money order, or cash) at the time of your physical examination. The checks and money orders should be made payable to: Salisbury State University.

If we do not receive this form, we will assume you are getting a physical exam by your own physician and a physical exam time will not be reserved for you here at SSU. You will be required to have a screening performed by an SSU certified athletic trainer. You must have your forms completed by your physician and they must be signed, stamped and/or notorized.

TIME

DATE

A specific time will be given to you, in advance, once we receive this form.

Konin JG, Frederick MA. *Documentation for Athletic Training*. Thorofare, NJ: SLACK Incorporated; 2005.

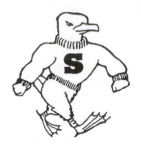

SALISBURY UNIVERSITY

Department of Intercollegiate Athletics, 1101 Camden Avenue
Salisbury, Maryland 21801-6860
www.salisbury.edu/athletics

Memo

To: **New & Transfer Athletes or Veterans Who Sat Out A Year**

From:

Subject: Physical Examinations

Included in this mailing is the yellow Health Screening Booklet and a reservation for a physical examination form. Your coach will contact you concerning times for Physical Examinations for your team and will contact you with your specific time. In order for us to plan appropriately we need your full cooperation. **YOU MUST RETURN TO US THE PHYSICAL EXAMINATION CONFIRMATION FOR IMMEDIATELY UPON RECEIVING IT.** This form and the booklet must be returned **immediately** indicating your desire to receive a physical here at SU. We will schedule physicals based on the forms returned. **If you do not return the forms no physical time or screening time will be allocated to you.** We will make a final schedule for the physicals and your coach will contact you with the exact time.

We highly recommend that you receive your physical here at SU. This allows for our physicians to meet you an initiates a relationship with the entire sports medicine staff. The cost of the physical will be $25. The checks or money orders can be made payable to Salisbury University. Cash will also be accepted. Sorry no credit cards will be accepted. If you choose to have your own personal physician perform your physical they must complete our forms and it must be stamped and/or notarized, **no exceptions**.

If you or your parents have any questions please contact me immediately. Your cooperation and quick response will enable us to plan efficiently and effectively. If your forms are not completed adequately the athletic training staff and the medical staff reserve the right to not allow your participation until adequate documentation is obtained. **Please read the entire Booklet first** and then complete the necessary information. The insurance information is extremely important. **Please supply us with a copy of your insurance card, both sides, when you return your information.**

Konin JG, Frederick MA. *Documentation for Athletic Training*. Thorofare, NJ: SLACK Incorporated; 2005.

HEALTH RECORD AND QUESTIONNAIRE
PARENT / GUARDIAN CONSENT

Pages 1-5 must be completed and signed by parent or guardian.

Date:_____

PERSONAL INFORMATION

Name_____Date of Birth_____Age on Last Birthday_____

Current Address _____

_____

Current Phone # (_____)_____

Resident of _____Public School District   Enrolled in_____School

Family Physician _____

Address and Phone #_____

_____

GENERAL INFORMATION

Does the student have or have a history of the following:

YES	NO		EXPLAIN
Y	N	Asthma	
Y	N	Diabetes	
Y	N	Heart Problems	
Y	N	Dizziness	
Y	N	Chest Pain/Angina	
Y	N	Extra Heart Beat	
Y	N	Blackouts/Loss of Consciousness	
Y	N	Rheumatic Fever	
Y	N	Cancer	
Y	N	Allergies	
Y	N	Medication	
Y	N	Food	
Y	N	Bites/Stings	
Y	N	High Blood Pressure	
Y	N	Drug or Alcohol Problems	
Y	N	Cysts or Lumps	
Y	N	Hepatitis	
Y	N	Heat Cramps/Exhaustion/Stroke	
Y	N	Skin Problems (itching, rashes, or acne)	
Y	N	Infectious Mononucleosis (Mono)	
Y	N	Loss of Paired Organ (i.e. eye, testicle)	

(Continued...)

Pennsylvania Department of Health • Governor's Council on Physical Fitness and Sports
January 2002/Revised July 2002

Name_____

YES	NO	EXPLAIN
Y	N	Does the student wear glasses or contact lenses?_____
Y	N	Does the student have any special protective equipment needs?_____
Y	N	Does the student take any medications?_____
		If so, over-the-counter, prescription, herbal, or dietary supplements? (circle all that apply)
		Medications:_____
Y	N	Has the student ever used anabolic steroids?_____
Y	N	Has the student ever used extreme measures to avoid weight gain or loss?_____
Y	N	Weight change in last six months? How Much _____ Up or down _____
Y	N	Has the student ever had surgery?_____
		If so, when and what?_____
Y	N	Has the student ever had varicella (chicken pox)?_____

When was the student's last tetanus shot?____Measles shot x 2_____Hepatitis B Vaccination x 3_____

ABDOMINAL

Does the student have or have a history of the following:

YES	NO	EXPLAIN
Y	N	Appendicitis_____
Y	N	Stomach Trouble_____
Y	N	Bleeding from Rectum_____
Y	N	Injury to Spleen_____
Y	N	Hernia_____
Y	N	Injury to Kidney_____

Are the following organs intact and normal as far as you know? Indicate absence of organs:

Y	N	Lungs_____
Y	N	Kidneys_____
Y	N	Testes_____
Y	N	Eyes_____
Y	N	Ears_____

NEUROLOGICAL

Does the student have or have a history of the following:

YES	NO	EXPLAIN
		Head Injury
Y	N	Skull Fracture_____
		How many concussions total?_____
Y	N	Concussion (memory loss, headache, confusion, nausea)_____
		Last concussion was_____months ago?
		How long did concussion last?_____

(Continued...)

Name_____

YES	NO		EXPLAIN

Y   N   Unconsciousness_____

How long did unconsciousness last? _____minutes/seconds.

Y   N   Neck Injury _____

Fracture _____

What spinal level?_____

Y   N   Pinched Nerve (Burner or Stingers)_____

Left_____or Right_____or Both _____

Y   N   Frequent Headaches _____

How often?_____

Y   N   Seizure Disorder_____

Y   N   Depression or Anxiety_____

EAR-NOSE-THROAT
Does the student have or have a history of the following:

YES	NO		EXPLAIN

Y   N   Hearing Difficulty _____

Y   N   Frequent Earaches_____

Y   N   Problems Breathing through Nose_____

Y   N   Broken Nose _____

Y   N   Frequent Tonsil Infections _____

Y   N   Cough after or during Exercise _____

DENTAL
Does the student have or have a history of the following:

YES	NO		EXPLAIN

Y   N   Cavities_____

Y   N   False Teeth_____

Y   N   Many Toothaches_____

Y   N   Missing Teeth_____

Y   N   Does the student Have A Dentist?_____

(Continued...)

Konin JG, Frederick MA. *Documentation for Athletic Training.* Thorofare, NJ: SLACK Incorporated; 2005.

Name_____

FEMALES

YES	NO		EXPLAIN
Y	N	Does the student have a history of an eating disorder._____	

First menstrual period was at age_____. Last menstrual period was_____ days ago.

The longest time between periods over the last year was_____months.

Periods last____days.

| Y | N | Is the student pregnant?_____ |

FAMILY HEALTH HISTORY

Has any member of the student's family died from or now have any of the following:

YES	NO		EXPLAIN (RELATION AND AGE)
Y	N	Died Suddenly_____	
Y	N	Heart Disease_____	
Y	N	Diabetes_____	
Y	N	High Blood Pressure_____	
Y	N	Seizure Disorder_____	
Y	N	Sickle Cell Trait/Disease_____	
Y	N	Has the student had any other medical conditions not listed?_____	
		If yes, explain_____	
		_____	

ORTHOPEDIC

Does the student have or have a history of any injury to any of the following? Please explain whether the injury was right or left, indicate the month and year of the injury, and if the student fully recovered from the injury:

YES	NO		EXPLAIN
		Cervical Spine	
Y	N	Fracture_____	
Y	N	Pinched Nerve_____	
Y	N	Stinger/Burner_____	
		Thoracic Region	
Y	N	Upper Back_____	
Y	N	Chest, Ribs_____	
		Lumbar Spine (Lower Back)	
Y	N	Muscle spasm, strain_____	
Y	N	Fracture or other_____	
Y	N	Shoulders_____	
Y	N	Upper Arm/Elbow_____	
Y	N	Forearm/Wrist_____	
Y	N	Hand/Fingers_____	
Y	N	Pelvis/Hip/Groin_____	
Y	N	Thigh: Quadriceps_____	

Pennsylvania Department of Health • Governor's Council on Physical Fitness and Sports
January 2002/Revised July 2002   36

(Continued...)

Name_____

YES	NO	EXPLAIN

Y N Hamstrings_____

Y N Other_____

Y N Knees_____

Y N Lower Leg/Ankle_____

Y N   Calf/Shin_____

Y N Achilles Tendon_____

Y N   Ankle_____

Y N Foot/Toes_____

Y N Diagnostic Tests: Bone Scan_____

CAT Scan_____

MRI Scan_____

X-Rays_____

Ultrasound_____

Other_____

Y N Has the student had any other injuries to bones, joints, muscles, or nerves (dislocations, tendinitis, calcium deposits, fractures, spurs, etc.) not listed herein?

If yes, explain _____

_____

_____

Y N **I certify that to the best of my knowledge all of the information herein is true and complete.**

Y N **I grant permission for medical personnel, at their discretion, to release my child's school health record medical information, including information from the Health Record and Questionnaire and physical evaluation, to those individuals deemed necessary by the medical personnel.**

Y N **I give my consent for the above-named student to commence practice and participate in athletic Contests during the _____ school year in the sport(s) of _____**

_____

Parent/Guardian Signature _____ Date___/___/____

PREPARTICIPATION SPORTS PHYSICAL EVALUATION

Must be completed and signed by medical personnel performing student's physical evaluation.

Name _____ Enrolled in_____ School

Sport _____ Age _____

Height_____ Weight_____ BP_____/_____ Pulse_____ Handed R_____ or L_____

Parent/Guardian_____ Phone_____

Family Physcian_____ Phone_____

Medical personnel performing physical evaluation for a student wrestler must complete the attached Minimum Wrestling Weight Classification form, which must set forth the minimum weight classification at which the student named herein, may wrestle for the entire season.

Medical Examination

Normal Abnormal Findings   **If Abnormal Explain**

Y	N	EENT_____
Y	N	Cardiovascular_____
Y	N	Cardiopulmonary_____
Y	N	Lungs _____
Y	N	Abdomen _____
Y	N	Genitourinary _____
Y	N	Neurological _____
Y	N	Skin _____
Y	N	Other_____

Musculoskeletal Exam

Y	N	Scoliosis _____
Y	N	Special Tests (Based on History Form) _____
Y	N	Neck _____
Y	N	Shoulder_____
Y	N	Elbow_____
Y	N	Wrist _____
Y	N	Hand_____
Y	N	Back _____
Y	N	Knee_____
Y	N	Ankle _____
Y	N	Foot _____
Y	N	Other_____

Clearance for sports participation:

A. Cleared

B. Cleared after completing evaluation / rehabilitation for: _____

C. Not Cleared for ☐ Collision ☐ Contact ☐ Noncontact ☐ Strenuous ☐ Moderately Strenuous ☐ Nonstrenuous

Due to: _____

_____

Recommendation/Referral: _____

_____

Name of Medical Examiner:_____ Date:_____

Address:_____ Phone_____

Signature MD, DO, PAC, CRNP, SNP _____

Pennsylvania Department of Health • Governor's Council on Physical Fitness and Sports
January 2002/Revised July 2002

Konin JG, Frederick MA. *Documentation for Athletic Training.* Thorofare, NJ: SLACK Incorporated; 2005.

Athlete Health Review

Name: _____   Sport: _____

Family History

Father: _____

Mother: _____

Siblings: _____

Other: _____

Allergies: _____

Past Surgical History:

_____

_____

_____

Past Medical History:

_____

_____

_____

Medication/Dose/Date(s)

_____   _____

_____   _____

_____   _____

Date/Current Problems

_____

_____

_____

_____

_____

_____

_____

_____

_____

_____

_____

_____

_____

_____

_____

_____

_____

_____

_____

_____

Konin JG, Frederick MA. *Documentation for Athletic Training*. Thorofare, NJ: SLACK Incorporated; 2005.

MEDICAL HISTORY QUESTIONNAIRE

TODAYS DATE_____

NAME:_____ Social Security #:_____
(full legal name)
Parent/Guardian Name:_____

Parent Home Address:_____

_____

City _____ State _____ Zip _____

Parent Home Phone:(__)_____ Parent Work Phone:(__)_____

Sport:_____ Age:_____ Single:____ Married:____ Date of Birth:_____

EMERGENCY NOTIFICATION: Name:_____

Relationship:_____ Telephone #(__)_____

Address:_____

City,State,Zip Code:_____

PERMISSION TO TREAT: Permission is given for the Athletic Training Services and Taylor Health Center to perform such examinations, immunizations, and medical tests as are deemed necessary and to administer such medical treatment as may be advisable to_____. I understand that the expenses incurred for medical care beyond that which is provided within Athletic Training Services are my responsibility.
Signed:_____ Signed:_____
Student/Athlete (Parent/Guardian, student under 18)

	If living Age Health	If Deceased Age at Death Cause	Has any relative ever had: (Circle)		WHO
Bio/Father			Cancer	Yes/No	
Bio/Mother			Tuberculosis	Yes/No	
Bio/Bro/Sis			Diabetes	Yes/No	
1.			Heart Trouble	Yes/No	
2.			High blood pressure	Yes/No	
3.			Stroke	Yes/No	
4.			Epilepsy	Yes/No	
			Mental Illness	Yes/No	

NOTE: This is a confidential record of your medical history and will be kept in this office. Information contained here will not be released to any person except when you have authorized us to do so. PLEASE CIRCLE ALL ANSWERS AND PROVIDE INFORMATION WITH ALL "YES" ANSWERS. ATTACH DOCUMENTS WHERE NECESSARY.

PERSONAL HISTORY
Illnesses: Have you ever had
Measles_____ No Yes
German Measles_____ No Yes
Mumps_____ No Yes
Chicken Pox_____ No Yes
Whopping Cough_____ No Yes
Scarlet Fever or Scarlatina____ No Yes
Diphtheria_____ No Yes
Smallpox_____ No Yes
Pneumonia_____ No Yes
Pleurisy_____ No Yes
Rheumatic fever or heart disease_ No Yes
Arthritis or Rheumatism_____ No Yes
Any bone or joint disease_____ No Yes
Neuritis or neuralgia_____ No Yes
Gonorrhea or Syphilis_____ No Yes
Gallbladder disease_____ No Yes
Anemia_____ No Yes
Jaundice_____ No Yes
Bladder Disease_____ No Yes
Eating Disorder(anorexia or
  bulimia)_____ No Yes
Epilepsy_____ No Yes
Migraine headaches_____ No Yes
Tuberculosis_____ No Yes
Diabetes_____ No Yes
Cancer_____ No Yes
Seizures_____ No Yes
Hepetitis A, B, C or D___ ____ No Yes
Colitis or other Bowel Disease___ No Yes
Hemorrhoids or any Rectal Disease No Yes
Nervous Breakdown_____ No Yes

Food, Chemical or Drug Poisoning_ No Yes
Asthma_____ No Yes
Exercise induced asthma_____ No Yes
Hives or Eczema_____ No Yes
Frequent Infections or Boils____ No Yes
Any Other Disease_____ No Yes
Allergies: Are you allergic to
Penicillin or Sulfa_____ No Yes
Aspirin, Codeine, or Morphine___ No Yes
Mycins or Other Antibiotics____ No Yes
Merthiolate or Mercurochrome____ No Yes
Any Other Drug_____ No Yes
Adhesive Tape_____ No Yes
Tape Adherent_____ No Yes
Nail Polish or Other Cosmetics___ No Yes
Tetanus Antitoxin or Serums____ No Yes
Other_____ No Yes
Weight: Now ___One Year Ago_____
  Maximum____When_____
Transfusions: Have you ever had
Blood or Plasma transfusion ___ No Yes
  Are you of African American or
Mediterranean decent:_____ No Yes
Have you had a sickle cell test__ No Yes

List all Surgeries you have had in the last 5 years.
_____
_____
_____
_____
_____

Have you ever been advised to have any surgical operation which has not been done?_____ No Yes
Have you been hospitalized for any illness?_____ No Yes
Give details_____
_____

INJURIES: Have you had (If yes, give specific dates and body parts)
Broken or cracked bones   No Yes
Sprains   No Yes
Lacerations   No Yes
Dislocations   No Yes
Concussion, or Head Injury   No Yes

(Continued...)

Konin JG, Frederick MA. *Documentation for Athletic Training*. Thorofare, NJ: SLACK Incorporated; 2005.

DO YOU NOW HAVE OR HAVE YOU HAD WITHIN THE PAST YEAR (If yes, please give specific details)

Frequent or severe headaches?	No / Yes
Fainting spells?	No / Yes
Unconscious spells?	No / Yes
Blurred vision?	No / Yes
Double vision?	No / Yes
Spots before eyes?	No / Yes
Infected eyes?	No / Yes
Pain behind eyes?	No / Yes
Any change in vision?	No / Yes
Do you wear glasses?	No / Yes
When were they last checked?	No / Yes
Do you wear contact lenses?	No / Yes
Hard?	
Soft?	
During competition?	No / Yes
Earaches?	No / Yes
Discharge from ears?	No / Yes
Ringing in ears?	No / Yes
Decrease in hearing?	No / Yes
Hearing problems?	No / Yes
Recurrent nose bleeds?	No / Yes
Recurrent head colds?	No / Yes
Sinus troubles?	No / Yes
Hay fever?	No / Yes
Strange or persistent odors?	No / Yes
Persistent hoarseness?	No / Yes
Difficulty swallowing ?	No / Yes
Enlarged glands?	No / Yes
Recurrent sore throats?	No / Yes
Recurrent sores in mouth?	No / Yes
Soreness or bleeding gums on brushing?	No / Yes
Chest pain?	No / Yes
Coughed up blood?	No / Yes
Pain in arm(s)?	No / Yes
Night sweats?	No / Yes
Chronic or frequent cough?	No / Yes
Chronic or frequent cough on lying down?	No / Yes
Wake up at night short of breath?	No / Yes
How many bed pillows do you use?	No / Yes
Shortness of breath on:	
Walking several blocks?	No / Yes
One flight of stairs?	No / Yes
On lying down?	No / Yes
Purple lips or fingers?	No / Yes
Palpitations or fluttering of heart?	No / Yes
High or low blood pressure?	No / Yes
Swelling of hands, feet, or ankles?	No / Yes
Dizziness with activity?	No / Yes
At what time of day?	
Details:	No / Yes
Leg cramps on waking or at night?	No / Yes
Enlarged veins in legs	No / Yes

(08/13/02)   Athlete's Name _____

Recurrent stomach pains?	No / Yes
Belching or heartburn?	No / Yes
Relieved by food or medication?	No / Yes
Appetite: Good Fair Poor	
Nausea or vomiting?	No / Yes
Avoid some foods?	No / Yes
What kinds?	
Avoid spices?	No / Yes
Abdominal cramps?	No / Yes
Change of color of bowel movements?	No / Yes
Change in size, shape, or texture of bowel movement?	No / Yes
Pain on urinating?	No / Yes
Difficulty in starting urination?	No / Yes
Do you get up at night to urinate?	No / Yes
How many times?	
Urinate more than before?	No / Yes
Urinate less than before?	No / Yes
Any blood in urine?	No / Yes
How many times per day do you urinate?	No / Yes
Full feeling of bladder, but only small amount upon urination?	No / Yes
Lose urine on coughing or sneezing?	No / Yes
Recurrent back pains?	No / Yes
Backaches?	No / Yes
Joint pains?	No / Yes
Swelling of any joints?	No / Yes
Redness or heat of any joint?	No / Yes
Tingling or weakness of hands or feet?	No / Yes
Muscle spasms?	No / Yes
Loss or change in sensation of hands or feet?	No / Yes
Trembling of any extremity?	No / Yes
Growth in neck or throat?	No / Yes
Hot flashes?	No / Yes
Tiredness without apparent reason?	No / Yes
Brittleness of nails?	No / Yes
Dryness of skin?	No / Yes
Easy bruising?	No / Yes
Inability to stand heat?	No / Yes
Inability to stand cold?	No / Yes
Change in hair texture?	No / Yes
Any skin rash?	No / Yes

X-RAYS: Have you ever had x-rays of:

Chest?	No / Yes
Stomach or colon?	No / Yes
Gall bladder?	No / Yes
Extremities?	No / Yes
Back?	No / Yes
Teeth?	No / Yes
Other (describe)?	No / Yes

EKG: Have you ever had an electrocardiogram?   No / Yes

IMMUNIZATIONS – Please give specific dates:

Diphtheria Tetanus	/ /	No / Yes
Polio		No / Yes
Measles (rubeola)	/ /	No / Yes
Mumps or MMR	/ /	No / Yes
Smallpox	/ /	No / Yes
Tuberculin skin test		No / Yes
Positive	Negative	
Other	/ /	No / Yes

IDENTIFY ANY MEDICATION(S) YOU ARE CURRENTLY TAKING:

☐ Accutane	☐ Midol	☐ Ventolin
☐ Advil	☐ Minocycline	☐ Xanax
☐ Albuterol	☐ Paxil	☐ Zantac
☐ Amoxicillin	☐ Proventil	☐ Zoloft
☐ Aspirin	☐ Ritalin	☐ Other:
☐ Atrovent	☐ Sudafed	
☐ Benadryl	☐ Sulfa Drugs	
☐ Ceclor	☐ Tagamet	
☐ Claritin	☐ Tavist	
☐ Ibuprofen	☐ Tetracycline	
☐ Keflex	☐ Tylenol	
☐ Klonopin	☐ Inhalers →	

Have you ever been treated for drug habits? _____ No / Yes

Have you ever taken insulin or tablets for diabetes? _____ No / Yes

Have you ever taken hormone tablets or injections? _____ No / Yes

WOMEN ONLY – MENSTURAL HISTORY

Regular? Yes No Varies	
Cycle – Days from start to start	
Flow: Heavy Medium Light	
Any clots passed?	No / Yes
Pains or cramps?	No / Yes
Date of last period?	
Date of last pelvic exam?	
Date of last Pap test?	
Results – Negative Positive	
Any discharge from vagina?	No / Yes
If so, color?	
Amount	
Any itching of vaginal area?	No / Yes
Do you take birth control pills?	No / Yes
Name?	
How long have you taken them?	

MEN ONLY

Discharge from penis? _____ No / Yes

Konin JG, Frederick MA. *Documentation for Athletic Training*. Thorofare, NJ: SLACK Incorporated; 2005.

Orthopedic History

ST. JOHN'S
Clinic - Orthopedic Specialists

The information requested below is important to your health.
Please answer all questions fully and accurately.

Date: _____

Patient's Legal Name: _____

_____
Last Name   First Name   Middle Initial

Date of Birth: _____ Age: _____ Are you <u>right</u> or <u>left</u> handed? Circle One

Name of person who sent you to our clinic: _____

_____
REASON FOR VISIT: My area of pain or complaint(s) is/are:

_____
What part of your body is experiencing the greatest pain?

Please rate the pain from 0 (no pain) to 10 (unbearable pain) _____

PAIN
☐   Sudden Onset: Since: _____
☐   Gradual Onset: Since: _____
☐   Onset Following an Injury: Since: _____

For Office Use Only

Vital Signs: BP _____
              Pulse _____
              Temp _____
              Resp _____

Height _____ Weight _____

Diagnosis(es) _____
_____
_____

X-ray views
_____
_____

- -

If applicable

Test dates _____
Return to clinic _____

PAST MEDICAL HISTORY (Conditions/problems you have had in the past)

( )Anemia (low blood count)   ( )Gout   ( )Mental Illness   ( )Prostate Problems   ( )Gallstones
( )Arthritis   ( )Heart Attack   ( )Rheumatic Fever   ( )Gastric Reflux   ( )Kidney Stones
( )Asthma   ( )Heart Trouble   ( )Seizures (convulsions) ( )Hiatal Hernia   ( )Tuberculosis
( )Cancer   ( )Hepatitis   ( )Stomach Ulcers   ( )Blood Clots   ( )Glaucoma
( )Cirrhosis   ( )High Blood Pressure ( )Sugar Diabetes   ( )Stroke   ( )Liver Disease
( )Emphysema   ( )Kidney Infection   ( )Thyroid Trouble   ( )Alcohol/Drug Abuse
( )Yellow Jaundice   ( )X-ray Exposure to Head or Neck (except chest x-ray).

PAST SURGICAL HISTORY Check the appropriate box and list the appropriate year?

( ) Appendix _____   ( ) Hernia, Hiatal _____
( ) Bypass _____   ( ) Hernia, Inguinal (groin) _____
( ) Cataracts _____   ( ) Hysterectomy _____
( ) Gallbladder _____   ( ) Stomach Ulcer _____
( ) Hemorrhoid _____   ( ) Tonsils/Adenoids _____
( ) Other _____

Spinal Surgery: ☐ Cervical Spine   ☐ Thoracic Spine   ☐ Lumbar Spine
                          Date:_____   Date: _____   Date: _____

MEDICATIONS Complete list below or present your list of all medications including herbs, vitamins, aspirin, etc.

_____ _____ _____ _____
_____ _____ _____ _____
_____ _____ _____ _____
_____ _____ _____ _____

MEDICATION ALLERGIES: _____
OTHER ALLERGIES: _____

Please see other side

(Continued...)

Konin JG, Frederick MA. *Documentation for Athletic Training*. Thorofare, NJ: SLACK Incorporated; 2005.

FAMILY HISTORY Please check the disease that runs in your family and indicate family member affected.

Mother (M)   Brother (B)   Aunt (A)
Father (F)   Child (C)   Uncle (U)
Sister (S)   Grandparents (GP)   Cousin (CS)

Example: Father and Brother with High Blood Pressure. (✔) HBP   <u>F, B</u>

( ) Bleeding Trouble _____   ( ) Heart Attack _____
( ) Breast Cancer _____   ( ) High Blood Pressure _____
( ) Colitis _____   ( ) Kidney Disease _____
( ) Diabetes _____   ( ) Tuberculosis _____
( ) Seizures (Epilepsy) _____ ( ) Ulcers _____
OTHER: _____

SOCIAL HISTORY
How often do you exercise? (please circle)   Daily   Weekly   Monthly   Rarely   Never
What type of exercise? _____
Approximate number of alcoholic beverages consumed <u>per week</u>: _____
Chew Tobacco   ( ) No   ( ) Yes
Smoke   ( ) No   ( ) Yes   How many packs? _____
                                                          Total number of years smoking: _____
Do you have a history of substance abuse? ( ) No ( ) Yes If so, what? _____
Education: Circle highest level: None <u>1 2 3 4 5 6 7 8</u> / <u>9 10 11 12</u> / <u>1 2 3 4</u>   Masters Ph.D. Other _____
                                      Elementary   High School   College

Occupation – Briefly list job and approximate years employed: _____

Martial Status: _____   Number of Children: _____ Do you live alone? _____

REVIEW OF SYSTEMS   (Indicate **present** problems)

Constitutional	☐ Fevers	☐ Night Sweats	☐ Weight Loss	☐ Night Pain
Musculoskeletal/Joints:	☐ Muscular Disease	☐ Arthritis	☐ Joint Pains	
Neurological:	☐ Headaches	☐ Migraines	☐ Seizure Disorder	☐ Stroke
Endocrine:	☐ Diabetes	☐ Thyroid Disease		
Hematology:	☐ Anemia	☐ Blood Clots	☐ Bleeding Problems	☐ Phlebitis
Urinary	☐ Blood in Urine	☐ Frequent Urination	☐ Trouble Starting Urination	
	☐ Painful Urination	☐ Prostate Disease	☐ Trouble Stopping Urination	
	☐ Kidney Disease	☐ Kidney Stones	☐ Loss of Bladder Control	
Respiratory:	☐ Asthma	☐ Bronchitis	☐ Emphysema	☐ COPD
	☐ Pneumonia	☐ Tuberculosis		
Cardiovascular:	☐ Chest Pain	☐ Shortness of Breath	☐ High Blood Pressure	
	☐ Palpitations	☐ Mitral Valve Prolapse	☐ Angina	
Reproductive:	☐ Infections	☐ Venereal Disease	☐ Herpes	☐ Impotence
Gastrointestinal:	☐ Stomach Ulcers	☐ Pancreatitis	☐ Gall Bladder Trouble	☐ Colitis
	☐ Blood in Stool	☐ Hiatal Hernia	☐ Liver Disease	
	☐ Jaundice	☐ Constipation	☐ Loss of Bowel Control	
Cancer:	☐ Lung	☐ Breast	☐ Colon	☐ Prostate
	☐ Skin	☐ Stomach	☐ Kidney	☐ Bone
Immunological:	☐ HIV Positive	☐ AIDS		
Psychiatric	☐ Depression	☐ Schizophrenia	☐ Mental Retardation	☐ Dementia
Women Only:	☐ Endometriosis	☐ Birth Control Pills		
	Are you Pregnant?	☐ Yes Due Date:		☐ No

All of the responses above are **complete and correct** to the best of my knowledge.

PATIENT SIGNATURE _____

DATE: _____

REVIEWED BY: _____

Konin JG, Frederick MA. *Documentation for Athletic Training*. Thorofare, NJ: SLACK Incorporated; 2005.

Name _____   Sport _____

Please check or circle the correct yes or no response, and add a detailed description to each question answered yes in the space provided. Please consult a sports medicine staff member with any questions you may have.

Medical History

1. How long has it been since your last complete health exam, other than an exam that was required for you to participate in sports? _____

<table>
<tr><td></td><td></td><td>Yes</td><td>No</td></tr>
</table>

2. Have you had a medical illness or injury since your last check up or sports physical? ____ ____

3. Are you currently taking any prescription or nonprescription (over the counter) medications or pills (including birth control pills, insulin, allergy shots or pills, asthma inhalers, vitamin or mineral supplements including iron, Tylenol, anti-inflammatories including aspirin, Advil, Aleve, Motrin or any over the counter supplements)? Please list below.   ____ ____

	Medication/Supplement	Dose	Frequency of Use
1.	_____	_____	_____
2.	_____	_____	_____
3.	_____	_____	_____
4.	_____	_____	_____
5.	_____	_____	_____

4. Do you have an allergy to any:

	Yes	No	Specify Allergy:
Drug or medicine (over the counter or prescribed)	____	____	_____
Foods	____	____	_____
Insects or animals	____	____	_____
Plants, grasses, pollen, dust or other environmental factors	____	____	_____
Other	____	____	_____

5. Have you ever had a rash or hives develop during or after exercise? Yes   No

6. Have you ever been diagnosed with any of the following medical conditions?

	Yes	No		Yes	No
Mononucleosis	____	____	Jaundice	____	____
Rubella (German Measles)	____	____	Stomach or intestinal ulcer	____	____
Chicken pox	____	____	Hernia	____	____
Repeated sinus infections	____	____	Eczema	____	____
Nose fracture	____	____	Psoriasis	____	____
Hearing defect or loss	____	____	Diabetes	____	____

(Continued...)

Konin JG, Frederick MA. *Documentation for Athletic Training*. Thorofare, NJ: SLACK Incorporated; 2005.

_____   Sport _____

	Yes	No		Yes	No
Recurrent ear infection	___	___	Sickle cell anemia/carrier	___	___
Epilepsy	___	___	Other anemia	___	___
Tumor, growth, cyst, cancer	___	___	Abnormal bleeding/clotting disorder	___	___
Over active thyroid	___	___	Blood clot or embolism	___	___
Under active thyroid	___	___	Leukemia or other blood disorder	___	___
Arthritis	___	___	Kidney injury	___	___
Marfan syndrome	___	___	Frequent urinary infections	___	___
Depression	___	___	Injury to liver or spleen	___	___
Other mental disorder	___	___	Hepatitis	___	___
Birth defect	___	___	Asthma	___	___
Eating disorder	___	___	Other medical condition/disorder	_____	

7. Were you born with two normal: **Yes   No**

     Eyes   ___ ___

     Ears

     Kidneys   ___ ___

8. Do you presently have the following skin problems:

     Rash

     Fungal infection   ___ ___

     Cold sore(s)   ___ ___

9. Have you ever had heat exhaustion/heat stroke/ sun stroke?   **Yes   No**

     If yes, please specify _____

10. During or after exercise, have you ever: **Yes   No**

     Been dizzy or light-headed?   ___ ___

     Passed out (fainted)?   ___ ___

     Had chest pain, discomfort or tightness?   ___ ___

     Found it more difficult to breath than usual?   ___ ___

     Had problems with coughing?   ___ ___

11. Have you ever been told that you have a heart murmur?   ___ ___

12. Have you ever had racing of your heart, irregular or skipped beats?   ___ ___

13. Have you ever been told by a doctor that you have/had:

     High blood pressure?   ___ ___

     Pericarditis, myocarditis, endocarditis (infections of the heart)? ___ ___

     Rheumatic fever?   ___ ___

     High cholesterol?   ___ ___

     Other heart or vascular problems? (please specify) _____

(Continued...)

Konin JG, Frederick MA. _Documentation for Athletic Training_. Thorofare, NJ: SLACK Incorporated; 2005.

Name _____   Sport _____

14. Have you ever had any medical tests for your heart (i.e. EKG, echocardiogram)?   Yes   No

    If yes, please specify: **Test**   **Date**

        1.   _____   _____

        2.   _____   _____

        3.   _____   _____

15. Have you ever had: **Yes   No**

    Bronchitis?   ____   ____

    Tuberculosis?   ____   ____

    Asthma?   ____   ____

    If yes to asthma: **Medication   Dose**   **Frequency of use**

        1.   _____   _____   _____

        2.   _____   _____   _____

        3.   _____   _____   _____

                                                        Yes   No

    Wheezing that starts during or just after exercise?   ____   ____

    Pneumothorax (collapsed lung)?   ____   ____

16. Have you ever had a concussion (injury to the head) with or without loss of consciousness?

                                                        ____   ____

    If yes, how many times? _____

17. Have you ever been knocked unconscious?   ____   ____

    How many times? _____

    What is the longest time that you have been unconscious due to a head injury? _____

18. Have you ever had any long term problems due to a head injury (e.g. memory loss headaches)?

    _____

19. Have you ever had numbness, tingling, or weakness in your: **Yes   No**

    Shoulders/arms/hands?   ____   ____

    Buttocks?   ____   ____

    Legs/feet?   ____   ____

20. Have you ever had a "burner" or "stinger" (an injury causing a sudden burning pain and numbness down the arm and/or hand)?   ____   ____

    If yes, how many times? _____

    How long did they last? _____

21. Have you ever had a seizure?   ____   ____

22. Do you experience migraine headaches?   ____   ____

    If yes, what medication do you take and how often? _____

(Continued...)

Konin JG, Frederick MA. *Documentation for Athletic Training*. Thorofare, NJ: SLACK Incorporated; 2005.

Name _____   Sport _____

	Yes	No
23. Have you ever had a serious eye injury?	___	___
If yes, please specify _____		
24. Do you wear glasses or contact lenses?	___	___
If yes:		
Do you wear glasses or contacts when you train or compete?	___	___
Have you had your eyes checked in the past 12 months?	___	___
25. Are you legally blind in either of your eyes?	___	___

WOMEN ONLY

26. At what age did your menstrual periods start? _____

27. When was your most recent menstrual period? _____

28. In the **past 12 months**:	Yes	No
Have you had trouble with heavy menstrual bleeding?	___	___
Have you had bleeding between periods?	___	___
Have you had menstrual cramps or pain that affected your school or athletic performance?	___	___
Have you had any unusual discharge from your vagina?	___	___
How many periods have you had? _____		
What was the longest time between periods? _____		
On average, how long has each period lasted? _____		

29. Are you presently taking any female hormones (estrogen, progesterone, birth control pills) for the purpose of regulating your periods?   ___ ___

30. Have you ever had a pelvic exam/Pap smear?   ___ ___

If yes:

When was your last pelvic exam/PAP smear? _____

Has your pelvic exam/PAP smear ever been abnormal?   ___ ___

MEN ONLY	Yes	No
31. Were you born with two normal testicles?	___	___
32. Have you ever had surgery to remove or repair a testicle (s)?	___	___
If yes, please specify _____		

SURGICAL HISTORY

33. Have you ever had surgery to the following:

	Yes	No	Date (mo/yr)	If yes, give reason for surgery
Brain	___	___	___/___	_____
Eyes	___	___	___/___	_____
Ears/nose/throat	___	___	___/___	_____
Heart	___	___	___/___	_____

(Continued...)

Konin JG, Frederick MA. *Documentation for Athletic Training.* Thorofare, NJ: SLACK Incorporated; 2005.

Name _____   Sport _____

	Yes	No	Date (mo/yr)	If yes, give reason for surgery
Lungs	____	____	___/___	_____
Stomach/bowels/appendix	____	____	___/___	_____
Kidneys	____	____	___/___	_____
Liver/spleen	____	____	___/___	_____
Bone	____	____	___/___	_____
Muscle/ligament/tendon	____	____	___/___	_____
Joint	____	____	___/___	_____
Other (please specify)			_____

FAMILY HISTORY

34. Please indicate if any of your full-blooded relatives listed below have a family history of the following:

	No history	Mother/Father	Brother/Sister	Grandparent
High blood pressure	_____	_____	_____	_____
Heart attack	_____	_____	_____	_____
Other heart abnormalities	_____	_____	_____	_____
(i.e.- hypertrophic cardiomyopathy, long QT syndrome, abnormal heart rhythm, etc.)				
High blood cholesterol	_____	_____	_____	_____
Diabetes	_____	_____	_____	_____
Arthritis	_____	_____	_____	_____
Bleeding disorder	_____	_____	_____	_____
Marfan syndrome	_____	_____	_____	_____
Kidney disease	_____	_____	_____	_____
Mental illness	_____	_____	_____	_____
Sickle cell anemia	_____	_____	_____	_____
Epilepsy	_____	_____	_____	_____
Cancer	_____	_____	_____	_____

35. Have any of your full-blood relatives died suddenly before the age of fifty, other than due to trauma? Please circle   **Yes**   **No**

     If yes, please specify _____

36. Please indicate your ethnic origin (circle all that apply)

    Native American/Alaska native   Hispanic/Latino/Chicano

    Asian   White (non Hispanic)

    Pacific Islander   Other, specify: _____

    Black/African American   Don't know

(Continued...)

Name _____   Sport _____

HEALTH HABITS

37. What is your current weight and height? _____

38. Are you happy with your current weight? _____

39. What would be your ideal weight? _____

40. Do you avoid eating any of the following:

	Yes	No
Meat?	____	____
Grains/bread?	____	____
Dairy?	____	____
Vegetables?	____	____
Fruits?	____	____
Any other food?	____	____

41. Have you ever been diagnosed with an eating disorder? ____ ____

42. Have you ever tried to control your weight with:

	Yes	No
Fasting?	____	____
Vomiting?	____	____
Laxatives?	____	____
Diuretics?	____	____
Diet pills?	____	____
Supplements?	____	____

43. Do you smoke? ____ ____

    If yes, how often and how many packs? _____

44. Do you use smokeless tobacco? ____ ____

45. Do you presently drink the following:

	Yes	No
Beer?	____	____
Wine or wine coolers?	____	____
Liquor?	____	____

    If yes, how often and how many drinks? _____

46. Have you used street drugs?

    If yes, how often and which drugs? _____

47. Have you ever sought treatment for or are you currently experiencing:

Anxiety/Stress?	____	____
Depression?	____	____
Mood Swings?	____	____
Hallucinations?	____	____
Sleep Disturbances?	____	____
ADHD/ Hyperactivity?	____	____

(Continued...)

Konin JG, Frederick MA. *Documentation for Athletic Training*. Thorofare, NJ: SLACK Incorporated; 2005.

Name _____   Sport _____

48. Have you ever tested positive for a communicable disease such as:

	Yes	No
Hepatitis C?	___	___
Hepatitis B?	___	___
Tuberculosis?	___	___
HIV?	___	___
Herpes (any form)?	___	___
Genital Warts?	___	___
Syphilis?	___	___

49. Do you use on a regular basis:

	Yes	No
Seat belts?	___	___
Bike helmet?	___	___

50. Have you ever been in an auto accident that resulted in personal injury?   **Yes**   **No**

ORTHOPEDIC HISTORY

51. In the past 12 months have you seen a physician, athletic trainer, physical therapist, chiropractor or other health care professional for a new or ongoing injury?   **Yes**   **No**

    If yes, please list the injury and specify if it has healed completely _____

    _____

    _____

    _____

52. Do you presently use for practice or competition:

	Yes	No
A brace, splint or sleeve?	___	___
Orthotics (shoe inserts)?	___	___
Neck roll?	___	___

Have you ever had or do you currently have an injury or problem with the following:

53. **Neck:**

	Yes	No		Yes	No
Disc disease	___	___	Facet disorder	___	___
Traumatic fracture	___	___	Surgery	___	___
Stress fracture	___	___	Other	___	___
Whiplash	___	___	specify: _____		

If yes:	Injury date (mo/yr)	Surgery date (mo/yr)	Current problems
1.	_____	_____	_____
2.	_____	_____	_____
3.	_____	_____	_____

(Continued...)

Konin JG, Frederick MA. *Documentation for Athletic Training*. Thorofare, NJ: SLACK Incorporated; 2005.

Name _____   Sport _____

54. Spine/Back:

	Yes	No		Yes	No
Congenital deformity/			Disc disease	___	___
Birth defect	___	___	Facet disorder	___	___
Traumatic fracture	___	___	Sacroiliac disorder	___	___
Stress fracture	___	___	Sciatica	___	___
Back pain	___	___	Scoliosis	___	___
Back stiffness	___	___	Surgery	___	___
Spondyloysis	___	___	Other	___	___
Spondylolisthesis	___	___	specify:	_____	

If yes: Injury date (mo/yr)   Surgery date (mo/yr)   Current problems

1.   _____
2.   _____
3.   _____

55. Shoulder/Clavicle:

	Yes	No		Yes	No	# of times
Traumatic fracture	___	___	Subluxation	___	___	_____
Bursitis	___	___	Dislocation	___	___	_____
Acromioclavicular (AC)	___	___	Surgery	___	___	
Separation	___	___	Instability	___	___	
Other	___	___	Rotator cuff tendonitis/			
Specify_____			impingement	___	___	

If yes: Injury date (mo/yr)   Surgery date (mo/yr)   Current problems

1.   _____   _____   _____
2.
3.   _____   _____   _____

56. Upper arm/forearm:

	Yes	No		Yes	No
Traumatic fracture	___	___	Surgery	___	___
Muscle injury	___	___	Other	___	___
Tendon injury	___	___	specify:	_____	

If yes: Injury date (mo/yr)   Surgery date (mo/yr)   Current problems

1.   _____   _____   _____
2.   _____   _____   _____
3.   _____   _____   _____

(Continued...)

Konin JG, Frederick MA. *Documentation for Athletic Training.* Thorofare, NJ: SLACK Incorporated; 2005.

Name _____   Sport _____

57. **Elbow:**

	Yes	No		Yes	No
Traumatic fracture	___	___	Dislocation	___	___
Ligament injury	___	___	Surgery	___	___
Tennis/golfer's elbow	___	___	Other	___	___
Bursitis	___	___	specify	_____	

If yes:	Injury date (mo/yr)	Surgery date (mo/yr)	Current problems
1.	_____	_____	_____
2.	_____	_____	_____
3.	_____	_____	_____

58. **Hand, wrist, fingers:**

	Yes	No		Yes	No
Traumatic fracture	___	___	Dislocation	___	___
Stress fracture	___	___	Surgery	___	___
Ligament injury	___	___	Other	___	___
Tendon injury or tendonitis	___	___	specify	_____	

If yes:	Injury date (mo/yr)	Surgery date (mo/yr)	Current problems
1.	_____	_____	_____
2.	_____	_____	_____
3.	_____	_____	_____

59. **Pelvis/Hip:**

	Yes	No		Yes	No
Traumatic fracture	___	___	Tendonitis	___	___
Stress fracture	___	___	Contusion/hip pointers	___	___
Groin strain	___	___	Surgery	___	___
Dislocation	___	___	Other	___	___
Bursitis	___	___	specify	_____	

If yes:	Injury date (mo/yr)	Surgery date (mo/yr)	Current problems
1.	_____	_____	_____
2.	_____	_____	_____
3.	_____	_____	_____

(Continued...)

Konin JG, Frederick MA. *Documentation for Athletic Training*. Thorofare, NJ: SLACK Incorporated; 2005.

Name _____   Sport _____

60. Thigh:

	Yes	No		Yes	No
Traumatic fracture	____	____	Quadriceps strain/injury	____	____
Stress fracture	____	____	Severe contusion	____	____
Tendonitis	____	____	Surgery	____	____
Bursitis	____	____	Other	____	____
Hamstring strain/injury	____	____	specify _____		

If yes:

	Injury date (mo/yr)	Surgery date (mo/yr)	Current problems
1.	_____	_____	_____
2.	_____	_____	_____
3.	_____	_____	_____

61. Knee:

	Yes	No		Yes	No	# of times
Meniscal injury	____	____	Swelling	____	____	
PCL tear	____	____	Dislocation of knee or patella			
			(knee cap)	____	____	_____
ACL tear	____	____	Pain around knee cap,			
Iliotibial band syndrome	____	____	(patello-femoral pain)	____	____	
Collateral ligament injury			Meniscal surgery	____	____	
(MCL, LCL)	____	____	Bursitis	____	____	
Tendonitis	____	____	ACL surgery	____	____	
Sensation of catching, instability, giving away, locking				____	____	
Other injury or surgery				____	____	
Specify _____						
Unexplained pain				____	____	
Specify _____						

If yes:

	Injury date (mo/yr)	Surgery date (mo/yr)	Current problems
1.	_____	_____	_____
2.	_____	_____	_____
3.	_____	_____	_____

(Continued...)

Name _____   Sport _____

62. **Lower leg:**

	Yes	No		Yes	No
Traumatic fracture	___	___	Shin splints	___	___
Stress fracture	___	___	Surgery	___	___
Muscle strain	___	___	Other	___	___
Compartment syndrome	___	___	specify _____		

If yes:

	Injury date (mo/yr)	Surgery date (mo/yr)	Current problems
1.	_____	_____	_____
2.	_____	_____	_____
3.	_____	_____	_____

63. **Ankle:**

	Yes	No		Yes	No
Traumatic fracture	___	___	Bone chip in joint	___	___
Stress fracture	___	___	Dislocation	___	___
Sprain	___	___	Surgery	___	___
Tendonitis	___	___	Bursitis	___	___
Instability	___	___	Other	___	___
			Specify _____		

If yes:

	Injury date (mo/yr)	Surgery date (mo/yr)	Current problems
1.	_____	_____	_____
2.	_____	_____	_____
3.	_____	_____	_____

64. **Foot/toes:**

	Yes	No		Yes	No
Traumatic fracture	___	___	Flat arches of feet	___	___
Stress fracture	___	___	Dislocation	___	___
Sprain	___	___	Surgery	___	___
Tendonitis/tendon injury	___	___	Neuroma	___	___
Bone spur	___	___	Plantar fascitis	___	___
Other	___	___			
Specify _____					

If yes:

	Injury date (mo/yr)	Surgery date (mo/yr)	Current problems
1.	_____	_____	_____
2.	_____	_____	_____
3.	_____	_____	_____

(Continued...)

Konin JG, Frederick MA. *Documentation for Athletic Training.* Thorofare, NJ: SLACK Incorporated; 2005.

Name _____   Sport _____

65. In the past 12 months, what is the total number of days of training and competition that you have been unable to participate in due to any injury?

	Never had	1-7 days	8-14 days	>14 days
Shin splints	_____	_____	_____	_____
Traumatic fracture (s)	_____	_____	_____	_____
Stress fracture (s)	_____	_____	_____	_____
Tendonitis or tendon injury (s)	_____	_____	_____	_____
Bursitis	_____	_____	_____	_____
Sprain	_____	_____	_____	_____
Pulled muscle (s)	_____	_____	_____	_____
Back problems (s)	_____	_____	_____	_____
Ligament injury or tear	_____	_____	_____	_____
Joint injury(s) or pain	_____	_____	_____	_____
Other injury_____	_____	_____	_____	_____
Other injury_____	_____	_____	_____	_____
Other injury_____	_____	_____	_____	_____

66. Have you ever had a cortisone injection into a tendon, bursa, or joint for an injury or pain?

If yes, please specify _____

_____

67. Are there any other injuries that have not been noted above that the University of Nevada should be aware of? _____

_____

_____

_____

_____

I acknowledge that all information above is correct and true to the best of my knowledge.

_____   _____
Print name   Date

_____
Athlete Signature

_____   _____
Parent/Guardian Signature if under 18   Date

Konin JG, Frederick MA. *Documentation for Athletic Training*. Thorofare, NJ: SLACK Incorporated; 2005.

James Madison University
Department of Sports Medicine
Health History Form
Academic Year 2004-05

Athlete's Name		Preferred Name	
Social Security #		Sport	
Email @jmu.edu		Phone #	

Allergies:

Agent	Yes	No	Specific Agent *and* Reaction
Medications			
Food			
Bee Stings			
Environmental			
Other			

Medications:

List all medications (including Over-the-Counter (OTC)) taken in the past 12 months for more than two weeks in a row (use reverse for additional medications if needed)

Medication	Current Use		Duration of Use
	Yes	No	

Surgical History

Please list all non-Orthopedic surgeries you have had (use if needed):

Nature of Surgery	Date

(Continued...)

Konin JG, Frederick MA. *Documentation for Athletic Training*. Thorofare, NJ: SLACK Incorporated; 2005.

Illness History:

Have you ever been told you have any of the following conditions in the past?

Condition	Yes	No	Condition	Yes	No	Condition	Yes	No
Anemia			Hypertension (high blood pressure)			Recurrent Urinary tract infection		
Arthritis			Hypoglycemia (low blood sugar)			Stomach Problem		
Asthma			Kidney stone			Substance abuse		
Bleeding Problem			Hepatitis or Liver disease			Thyroid problem		
Cancer			Lung disease			Seizures		
Diabetes			Migraines			Sexually Transmitted Disease		
Eye Problems			Ovarian Cyst			Syncope (fainting)		
Hearing loss			Rheumatic fever			Other		
HIV			Single kidney					
Hernia			Single testis					

In the space provided answer the following questions. Provide as much detail as possible (dates, treatment, tests) for all positive responses *(use reverse if needed)*:

Do you have any known heart condition?	
Have you ever been told you have a heart murmur?	
Have you ever been told you have an eating disorder?	
Where you ever told you have infectious mononucleosis (mono)	
Do you wear any type of dental appliance?	
Do you wear glasses or contacts? Do you wear them to compete?	
Are you under the care of a doctor for any chronic conditions?	
Have you gained or lost more than 10 pounds in the past year?	
Have you ever been told you have Sickle Cell trait?	
Have you ever been involved in a motor vehicle accident?	

(Continued...)

Konin JG, Frederick MA. *Documentation for Athletic Training*. Thorofare, NJ: SLACK Incorporated; 2005.

Female athletes only	
When was your first menstrual cycle?	
When was your last menstrual cycle?	
Since your cycles began have you gone for more than 4 months with a cycle?	
What is the typical interval between your cycles?	
What is the typical duration of your cycles?	
Do you experience significant pain or cramping with your cycles?	
When was your last PAP smear?	
Do you take oral contraceptives?	

Injury History:

Have you had any of the following injuries?

Condition	Yes	No	Condition	Yes	No	Condition	Yes	No
Ankle Sprain			Muscle Strain			Joint Dislocation		
Back Pain			Stress Fracture			Rotator Cuff Injury		
Bursitis			Tendon or Ligament Injury			Shin Splints		
Joint Instability			Tendonitis			Bone Spur or Chip		
Knee Injury			Fracture			Joint Separation		

For all questions with a Yes response, please provide details of this injury below:

Injury	Date	Treatment

(Continued...)

Konin JG, Frederick MA. *Documentation for Athletic Training*. Thorofare, NJ: SLACK Incorporated; 2005.

In the space provided answer the following questions. Provide as much detail as possible (dates, treatment, tests) for all positive responses *(use reverse if needed)*:

Have you ever had joint exploration, reconstruction or arthroscopic surgery?	
Have you ever had an injury resulting in you missing more than 1 week of games, practices. Or general participation?	
Have you ever had a joint, tendon or bursa injection or aspiration?	
Do you presently use a brace or splint for practice or competition?	
Have you ever had heat stroke, heat exhaustion or heat cramps?	
Have you ever had a concussion or head injury?	
Have you ever had a neck injury?	
Has any doctor ever recommended you not participate in athletics?	

(Continued...)

Konin JG, Frederick MA. *Documentation for Athletic Training*. Thorofare, NJ: SLACK Incorporated; 2005.

Health Habits:

Please answer the following questions as completely as possible in the space provided
(use reverse if needed)

What in your opinion would be your ideal body weight?		
Are there any foods you avoid eating? (check all that apply)	Meat	
	Bread/Grains	
	Dairy Products	
	Vegetables	
	Fruits	
	Other (specify)	
Do you smoke? If yes when did you start? How much do you smoke now?		
Do you use smokeless tobacco?		
How often do you consume alcoholic beverages? How much?		
When was your last drink?		
Have you ever used street drugs?		
Have you ever used anabolic steroids?		
Do you use herbal preparations of any kind? If so, what?		
Do you currently use supplements of any type? If so, what?		
Do you have problems sleeping? If so, please describe.		
Have you had any times of prolonged sadness or depression? If so, please describe		

(Continued...)

Konin JG, Frederick MA. *Documentation for Athletic Training.* Thorofare, NJ: SLACK Incorporated; 2005.

Family History:

Have any members of your family (parents, siblings, grandparents, aunts/uncles or cousins) had any of the following conditions?

Condition	Yes	No
Heart attack before the age of 50 (male) or 60 (female)		
Angioplasty or Bypass Surgery before 50 (male) or 60 (female)		
Sudden or Unexplained death?		
Collapse during physical activity		
Hypertension (High blood pressure)		
Heart Murmur or valve replacement		
Marfan's syndrome		
Seizures or Epilepsy		
Asthma or other lung disease		
Sickle Cell Disease		
Diabetes		
Depression		

_____
Athlete's Signature

_____
Date

If Athlete is under 18 year of age:

_____
Parent's Signature

_____
Date

Konin JG, Frederick MA. *Documentation for Athletic Training*. Thorofare, NJ: SLACK Incorporated; 2005.

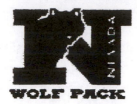

University of Nevada
Recruiting Physical Exam

Name_____ Sex_____ Age_____ Date of Birth_____

Sport_____ Height_____ Weight_____

Parents/Guardian Name and Phone _____

_____

Family History   Yes   No

1. Have you had a medical illness or injury since your last check up or sports physical? _____   _____

2. Have you ever been advised by a doctor "Not" to participate in any sport activity?   _____   _____

    If yes, why? _____

3. Have you ever had a chronic illness that lasted longer than one week or caused you to miss practice

    or event/game(s)?   _____   _____

    If yes, what? _____

4. Have you ever had surgery, or have you ever been advised to have surgery at any

    time in your life?   _____   _____

    If yes: What body Part?   When?

                1._____   _____

                2._____   _____

                3._____   _____

5. Do you have any allergies (for example: to pollen, medicine, food, or stinging insects? _____ _____

    If yes, please specify_____

6. Do you have any loss or impairment of organs (kidneys, eyes, testicles, lungs,   _____ _____

    ears, ovaries)? If yes, please specify_____

7. Do you currently have or have you ever had a tumor, growth, cyst or cancer?

    If yes, please specify_

8. Have you ever had a seizure or any altered brain function?   _____   _____

    If yes, please specify_____

9. Have you ever been told you have Marfan syndrome?   _____   _____

(Continued...)

Konin JG, Frederick MA. *Documentation for Athletic Training.* Thorofare, NJ: SLACK Incorporated; 2005.

	Yes	No

10. Have you ever been diagnosed with asthma? _____ _____

   If yes, what medications do you take?_____

11. During or after exercise, have you ever:

   Become ill from exercising in the heat? _____ _____

   Been dizzy or light-headed? _____ _____

   Passed out (fainted)? _____ _____

   Had chest pain, discomfort or tightness? _____ _____

   Found it more difficult to breathe than normal? _____ _____

   Had problems with coughing? _____ _____

12. Have you ever had racing of your heart or skipped heartbeats? _____ _____

13. Have you ever had high blood pressure or high cholesterol? _____ _____

14. Have you ever been told you have a heart murmur? _____ _____

15. Have you ever received treatment for your heart murmur? _____ _____

16. Has a physician ever denied or restricted your participation in sports for any heart _____ _____

   problems?

17. Have you ever been diagnosed with diabetes? _____ _____

   If yes, do you take insulin?_____

18. Have you ever had surgery or been told you need surgery to the following:

   Eyes? _____ _____

   Ears/Nose/Throat _____ _____

   Heart? _____ _____

   Lungs? _____ _____

   Stomach or bowels/appendix? _____ _____

   Kidneys? _____ _____

   Liver? _____ _____

   Spleen? _____ _____

   If yes, when?_____

19. Do you have a history of any of the following medical illnesses? (Circle the illness and explain)

   Seizure, Anemia, Diabetes, Tuberculosis, Arthritis, Thyroid Disease, Hepatitis (Jaundice),

   Infectious Mononucleosis, Hypertension (High Blood Pressure), Pneumonia, Rectal Pain or

   Bleeding, or other infectious disease?

   If yes, please explain_____

(Continued...)

Konin JG, Frederick MA. *Documentation for Athletic Training*. Thorofare, NJ: SLACK Incorporated; 2005.

20. Please indicate if any of your **full-blooded relatives** listed below have a family history of the following:

	No history	Mother/Father	Brother/Sister	Grandparent
High blood pressure				
Heart attack				
Other heart abnormalities				
High blood cholesterol				
Diabetes				
Arthritis				
Bleeding Disorder				
Marfan Syndrome				

Orthopedic History

                                                                                Yes No

21. Have you ever had a head injury or concussion (loss of consciousness, fainting, ____ ____

knocked out, or dinged within the last three years)?

        If yes, when?_____

22. Have you ever had an injury to the neck (Stinger, burner or pinched nerve)? ____ ____

23. Have you ever broken, fractured, or dislocated any joints? ____ ____

If yes:	What body part?	When?	How many times?
1.			
2.			
3.			

24. Have you ever strained or "pulled" a muscle? ____ ____

        If yes, what muscle and when?_____

25. Have you had any other problems with pain or swelling in muscles, ____ ____

tendons, bones or joints?

26. Have you ever had surgery or ever been told you need to have surgery on bone, muscle, ligament,

tendon, joint or any other body part? ____ ____

        If yes, please specify_____

27. Do you have any previous injuries that have now "healed"? ____ ____

        If yes, please explain_____

28. Have you had any of the following? (Circle)

        Stress fracture, Chondromalacia, Osgood Schlater's Disease, Little League Elbow, Shoulder

        Impingement, Arthritis, or Jumper's Knee

            If yes, are you currently having problems?_____

(Continued...)

Konin JG, Frederick MA. *Documentation for Athletic Training*. Thorofare, NJ: SLACK Incorporated; 2005.

29. Have you ever had a problem with: Yes   No

    Shoulder subluxation/dislocation?   ____ ____

    Shoulder impingement?   ____ ____

    Knee- ACL tear or sprain?   ____ ____

    Knee- patella subluxation/dislocation?   ____ ____

    Ankle sprains?   ____ ____

    Low back pain w/practice, weights and/or conditioning?   ____ ____

    Elbow pain?   ____ ____

30. Have you ever been to a physical therapist?   ____ ____

31. Have you ever been to a chiropractor?   ____ ____

32. Are there any other medical conditions that the University of Nevada should be aware of?

    Please explain _____

    _____

    _____

    _____

Comments (ATC only): _____

_____

_____

_____

_____

_____

_____

_____

_____

_____

_____

_____

_____

_____

_____

_____

_____

Athletic Trainer Signature: _____   **Date:** _____

Konin JG, Frederick MA. *Documentation for Athletic Training*. Thorofare, NJ: SLACK Incorporated; 2005.

James Madison University
Department of Sports Medicine

<u>Medical Recruitment History</u>

Name:		Sport:	
Address:			
City:		State:	Zip:
Phone:		Email:	

The NCAA allows athletes who are being recruited by an institution to undergo a medical screen by the Sports Medicine Department while on a campus visit in accordance with NCAA Bylaw 13.12.2.5. Completion of this form will assist James Madison University in evaluating your current medical history. Please respond to the questions as completely and accurately as possible. **If you have any questions you may contact the Department of Sports Medicine at (540) 568-6562.**

Do any of the following apply to you	Yes	No	Please explain in detail, including dates
Experienced episodes of dizziness, fainting, or passing out?			
Had a concussion?			
Had a neck injury (strain, stinger, burner, or disc problems, etc…)?			
Born with or acquired any impairment to organs (eyes, kidney, heart, etc…)?			
Been hospitalized, visited the emergency room, or had surgery?			
Been told you have high blood pressure or any other heart condition?			
Been told you have respiratory illnesses such as asthma, breathing difficulties?			
Have relatives experiencing sudden death prior to age 50 by natural causes?			
Ever experienced heat-related illnesses such as dehydration, heat exhaustion, heat stroke, heat cramps, etc…?			
Currently use any prescription medication on a regular basis to regulate any body systems (insulin, pain)?			
Do you require any special equipment that allows you to participate in sport (braces, orthotics, etc…)?			
Currently not participating in a sport due to an injury of any kind?			
Had any muscle, bone or joint injuries that have not required medical care?			
Had an eating or nutritional disorder?			
Ever tested positive on a drug test/screen			

I acknowledge that the above information is factual to the best of my knowledge, and that by signing below I grant permission to the JMU Sports Medicine Staff to share the above information with JMU coaches as deemed necessary.

_____   _____   _____   _____
Prospective Athlete   Date   Parent (if athlete under age 18)   Date

Konin JG, Frederick MA. *Documentation for Athletic Training*. Thorofare, NJ: SLACK Incorporated; 2005.

Recruiting Physical Evaluation Form

Lumbar Spine			**Comments**
Observation	**Norm**	**Abnorm**	
ASIS alignment			
PSIS alignment			
Lordosis			
Scoliosis			
Spondylolisthesis			

Lumbar Spine			**Comments**
ROM & Strength	**Norm**	**Abnorm**	
Flexion/Extension			
Lateral flexion			
Rotation (L/R)			

Special Tests	**Norm**	**Abnorm**	
Straight leg raise			
Gaenslen's Test			
Patrick Test			
Beevors Sign			

Hip and Pelvis			**Comments**
ROM & Strength	**Norm**	**Abnorm**	
Hip Flexion/Extension			
Hip Abduction/Adduction			
Hip Int./Ext. Rotation			
Flex./Ext. (knee bent)			

Special Tests	**Norm**	**Abnorm**	
Trendelenburg			
Ober Test			

Knee			**Comments**
Special Tests	**Norm**	**Abnorm**	
Apprehension			
Patellar Grind			
Lachman			
Anterior Drawer			
Posterior Laxity			
Valgus 0* & 30*			
Varus 0* & 30*			
McMurray's			

Ankle			**Comments**
Special Tests	**Norm**	**Abnorm**	
Plantar/Dorsi Flexion			
Inversion/Eversion			
Ant. Drawer (knee bent)			
Extensor Hallicus			
Talar Tilt			

(Continued...)

Konin JG, Frederick MA. *Documentation for Athletic Training.* Thorofare, NJ: SLACK Incorporated; 2005.

Recruiting Physical Evaluation Form

Neck			Comments
ROM &Strength	**Norm**	**Abnorm**	
Flexion			
Extension			
Lateral Flexion			
Rotation			
Special Tests	**Norm**	**Abnorm**	
Spurlings			
Adson			
Biceps Reflex (C5)			
Shoulder			**Comments**
ROM & Strength	**Norm**	**Abnorm**	
Flexion/ Extension			
Abduction/Adduction			
Int & Ext Rotation			
Horizontal Abd/Add			
Scaular Elevation			
Winging Scapula			
Special Tests	**Norm**	**Abnorm**	
Apprehension			
Empty Can Test			
Speeds Test			
Anterior Stability			
Posterior Stability			
Elbow			**Comments**
ROM & Strength	**Norm**	**Abnorm**	
Flexion/Extension			
Pronation/Supination			
Special Tests	**Norm**	**Abnorm**	
Valgus Stress			
Varus Stress			
Tinel sign			
Wrist & Hand			**Comments**
ROM & Strength	**Norm**	**Abnorm**	
Flexion/Extension			
Pronation/Supination			
Grip			
Finger Prehension			
Opposition			
Mallet/Boutonniere Deformity			

Konin JG, Frederick MA. *Documentation for Athletic Training*. Thorofare, NJ: SLACK Incorporated; 2005.

RECERTIFICATION FOR SPORTS PARTICIPATION

INTERIM HEALTH HISTORY
(to be completed by parent or guardian)

Date_____   FR/SOPH/JR/SR
                                                         (circle one)

PERSONAL INFORMATION

Name _____ Enrolled in_____School

Sport _____Age_____

Home Address_____ Phone _____

_____

Parent/Guardian _____ Phone _____

Family Physician _____ Phone _____

Within the past year has the student had:

YES	NO		EXPLAIN
Y	N	Any injury related to sports _____	
Y	N	Any injuries not related to sports _____	
Y	N	Any operations_____	
Y	N	Any illness requiring student to stay home or be hospitalized _____	
Y	N	Experienced dizzy spells or blackouts or unconsciousness_____	
Y	N	Any episodes of unexplained shortness of breath, wheezing, or chest pain_____	
		_____	
Y	N	Developed any new health problems_____	
Y	N	Any new medications, prescription or over the counter _____	
Y	N	Any health problems student wants to discuss with a doctor_____	

_____   _____
Parent/Guardian Signature   Date

Must be completed and signed by medical personnel performing student's recertification

Height_____ Weight_____ BP_____/_____ Pulse_____ Handed R_____ or L_____

Clearance for sports participation:

A. Cleared

B. Cleared after completing evaluation / rehabilitation for: _____

C. Not Cleared for ☐ Collision ☐ Contact ☐ Noncontact ☐ Strenuous ☐ Moderately Strenuous ☐ Nonstrenuous

Due to: _____

Recommendation/Referral: _____

Name of Examiner:_____ Date:_____

Address:_____ Phone:_____

Signature MD/DO, PAC, CRNP, SNP _____

Pennsylvania Department of Health • Governor's Council on Physical Fitness and Sports
January 2002/Revised June 2002

SMS ATHLETIC TRAINING SERVICES DEPARTMENT
Student-Athlete Recertification Physical Examination

Name _____   Social Security # _____

Date of Birth _____   Sport(s) _____

Since your last physical examination on _____, have you?
DATE

☐ Yes ☐ No	1. Had a serious injury / been hospitalized?	☐ Yes ☐ No	21. Had an unfavorable / allergic reaction to a drug, antibiotic, and/or medicine?
☐ Yes ☐ No	2. Had a severe sprain / strain and/or fracture?	☐ Yes ☐ No	22. Do you have only one of two paired, functioning organs (eye, kidney, ovary, etc.)?
☐ Yes ☐ No	3. Had a concussion and/or head injury?	☐ Yes ☐ No	23. Do you have any allergies?
☐ Yes ☐ No	4. Been unconscious for any other reason other than anesthesia?	☐ Yes ☐ No	24. Do you require daily medications?
☐ Yes ☐ No	5. Had a neck and/or back injury?	☐ Yes ☐ No	25. Been diagnosed with asthma?
☐ Yes ☐ No	6. Had a back injury or back pain?	☐ Yes ☐ No	26. Experienced wheezing?
☐ Yes ☐ No	7. Had a history of burners, stingers, numbness in neck, shoulder, and/or hand?	☐ Yes ☐ No	27. Been diagnosed with diabetes?
☐ Yes ☐ No	8. Had a shoulder, elbow, and/or hand/wrist injury?	☐ Yes ☐ No	28. Been diagnosed with kidney disease?
☐ Yes ☐ No	9. Had a hip and/or knee injury?	☐ Yes ☐ No	29. Been diagnosed with a hernia?
☐ Yes ☐ No	10. Had a lower leg, ankle, and/or foot injury?	☐ Yes ☐ No	30. Experienced seizures or convulsions; and/or been diagnosed with epilepsy?
☐ Yes ☐ No	11. Had an operation?	☐ Yes ☐ No	31. Been diagnosed with high blood pressure and/or high blood cholesterol?
☐ Yes ☐ No	12. Are you currently undergoing physical therapy or rehabilitation for an injury?	☐ Yes ☐ No	32. Do you require any special equipment to participate in athletics?
☐ Yes ☐ No	13. Do you have any medical problems about which we should be aware?	☐ Yes ☐ No	33. Have you been told by a physician to restrict your activity or not to participate in sport?
☐ Yes ☐ No	14. Do you wear contact lenses, glasses, and/or safety glasses?	☐ Yes ☐ No	34. Are you currently taking any short course medication for any illnesses?
☐ Yes ☐ No	15. Had frequent headaches?	☐ Yes ☐ No	35. Do you have any ongoing or chronic illnesses?
☐ Yes ☐ No	16. Had a heat related illness (heat cramps, heat exhaustion, and/or heat stroke)?	☐ Yes ☐ No	36. Have you had a history of anorexia, bulimia (forced vomiting), and/or any other eating disorder?
☐ Yes ☐ No	17. While exercising, has your heart ever "skipped" a beat, have you suffered from a "racing heart", severe chest pain, lightheadedness, or fainted?	☐ Yes ☐ No	37. Do you take vitamins, amino acids, creatine, and/or any other dietary supplement?
☐ Yes ☐ No	18. Had a dental injury?	☐ Yes ☐ No	38. Do you know of, or do you believe there is any health reason why you should not participate in intercollegiate athletics at SMS?
☐ Yes ☐ No	19. Do you wear a removable dental appliance?	☐ Yes ☐ No	39. Had trouble with coughing, wheezing, or breathing during or after exercise?
☐ Yes ☐ No	20. Been recently diagnosed with infectious mononucleosis ("mono"), hepatitis B or C, HIV/AIDS, and/or any other severe infectious disease / viral infection?	☐ Yes ☐ No	40. Have you ever felt dizzy or passed out during or after exercise

FEMALES ONLY!
When did your last menstrual period begin? _____
How long does your menstrual period usually last? _____
How many menstrual periods have you had in the last 12 months? _____
Do you take birth control pills? If so, which one(s)? _____
Do you take pain medication? If so, which one(s)? _____

If you answered "YES" to any of the above questions and/or have any further information, which is knowledgeable to you not required on this form, please explain in detail (use additional sheet(s) if necessary)-

I, the undersigned, hereby acknowledge, affirm, and represent that all above statements are true and accurate to the best of my knowledge; and that no answer information have been withheld. If any information and/or statements are false and/or have been omitted in reference to my past and/or present medical history understand that Southwest Missouri State University, its agents, servants, trustees, and employees disclaim liability, and will not be held liable for any injuries a illnesses not noted.

_____   _____
Student-Athlete Signature   Date

3/31/04

Konin JG, Frederick MA. *Documentation for Athletic Training*. Thorofare, NJ: SLACK Incorporated; 2005.

University of Nevada
STUDENT ATHLETE YEARLY PARTICIPATION PHYSICAL UPDATE

Date:_____

Name:_____ Sport:_____

Address:_____ City:_____ State:_____ ZIP:_____

DOB:_____ SS#:_____ Local Phone#:_____

Eligibility Year: 1 2 3 4 5   Year in School: FR SO JR SR 5th Year

Current medicaitons including prescription, over the counter and vitamins/minerals/suppliments

_____

Do you have any chronic pain? _____Yes _____No   From last season/year _____

      From Summer_____

Did you have any injuries over the summer? Yes_____   No_____

Please explain Yes answers: _____

_____

_____

Did you see a doctor and/or have any treatment over the summer? Yes_____   No_____

Please explain Yes answers: _____

_____

Did you have any medical problems or injuries during the last season? Yes_____   No_____

_____Head _____Neck _____Shoulder _____Forearm _____Wrist _____Hand

_____Chest _____Back _____Hip _____Thigh _____Knee _____Shin/Calf _____Ankle

_____Foot _____Illness _____Other

Do you have any concerns regarding these injuries or problems listed above? Yes_____   No_____

Please Explain:_____

_____

_____

HT_____   WT_____   BP_____/_____   Pulse_____

Athlete's Signature:_____   Date_____

Athletic Trainer's Signature:_____   Date_____

Konin JG, Frederick MA. *Documentation for Athletic Training*. Thorofare, NJ: SLACK Incorporated; 2005.

<u>Please read the following consent/authorization forms carefully:</u>
(If you are under 18 years of age, your parents must also sign)

The basic consent of each is:

A.	<u>Medical Consent:</u>	Allows the athletic trainers and team physician(s) to treat any injury you receive while at the University of Nevada.
B.	Authorization/Consent <u>To Disclose Information:</u>	Allows those listed to release information to the NCAA, Conference, media and professional teams concerning your injuries/illness.
C.	<u>Shared Responsibility</u> <u>for sport safety</u>	Acknowledges you that there are certain inherent risks involved in participating in intercollegiate athletics and that you are willing to assume responsibility for such risks.
D.	<u>Aids & Intercollegiate</u> <u>Athletics:</u>	Acknowledges that HIV transmission is possible through athletics.

If you should chose to refuse to sign any of these, please write **"Refuse to Sign"**, the date, and your signature.

A photo copy of these authorizations shall be considered as effective and valid as the original for the time I am a participant in the intercollegiate athletic program at the University of Nevada.

<u>FORMS</u>

A.   <u>Medical Consent</u>

I hereby grant permission to the University of Nevada team physician(s) and/or the consulting physician(s) to render to my son, daughter, or myself, any treatment or medical or surgical care that they deem reasonably necessary to the health and well being of the student athlete, including consults/referrals to outside medical professionals.

I also hereby authorize the athletic trainers at the University of Nevada who are under the direction and guidance of the University of Nevada team physician(s) to render to my son, daughter, or myself any preventative first aid, rehabilitation, or emergency treatment that they deem reasonably necessary to the health and well being of the student athlete.

In case of serious injury or illness, I understand that reasonable effort will be made to contact the parents/guardians. If contact cannot be made, I hereby give permission to the University of Nevada sports medicine staff, other facilities, or health care providers to administer emergency medical treatment including surgery as deemed advisable.

(Continued...)

Konin JG, Frederick MA. *Documentation for Athletic Training*. Thorofare, NJ: SLACK Incorporated; 2005.

I authorize the University of Nevada intercollegiate athletic department to provide the University of Nevada health center any information requested, and authorize the University of Nevada student health center to provide the University of Nevada intercollegiate athletic department any information requested, concerning my health and athletic status.

Also, when necessary for executing such case, I grant permission for hospitalization at an accredited hospital.

I understand and agree that the University of Nevada may use or disclose protected health information for treatment, payment and operations in accordance with the Notice of Privacy Practices that I have received, and any posted amendments to that Notice. I understand that the University of Nevada will not use or disclose protected health information for any purpose other than treatment, payment and healthcare operations, unless such person or entity is authorized to receive such information under law or I have provided a written authorization. (*See full explanation of disclosures and rights in the Notice of Privacy* **Practices**) If I am being treated while I am a student athlete, I consent and agree that my health information may be used and disclosed in accordance with the Notice of Privacy Practices (and any posted revision of that Notice) and the federal Health Insurance Portability and Accountability Act (HIPAA).

Date:_____   _____
                                                         Signature

Signature may be that of athlete 18 years   _____
of age and over: if under 18, please
have parent or guardian sign.   Social Security Number

                                                         _____
                                                         Parent or Guardian

B.   Consent/Authorization for Disclosure of Information

I, _____, hereby authorize _____
         Name of Student Athlete   Name of My Institution

and its coaches, physicians, athletic trainers and health care personnel to disclose my protected health information and any related information regarding any injury or illness during my training for, and participation in, intercollegiate athletics to the NCAA, my institution's athletic conference, to media outlets (including the University of Nevada Sports Information Office), to professional sports teams, and to their respective employees or agents.

(Continued...)

I understand that my protected health information will be used by the NCAA, Conference, media, and/or professional sports teams for the purpose of statistical reporting, providing to the public information regarding the general type of any injury or illness that I have incurred, the medical professionals involved in my care, the current status of my health, and my probable return date to active participation, and providing professional sports teams with medical/health information and records for player evaluation purposes.

I understand that my injury/illness information is protected by federal regulations under either the Health Information Portability and Accountability Act (HIPAA) or the Family Educational Rights and Privacy Act of 1974 (the Buckley Amendment) and may not be disclosed without either my authorization under HIPAA or my consent under the Buckley Amendment. I understand that my signing of this authorization/consent is voluntary and that my institution will not condition any health care treatment or payment, enrollment in a health plan or receipt of any benefits (if applicable) on whether I provide the consent/authorization requested. I also understand that I am not required to sign this authorization/consent in order to be eligible to participate in NCAA or conference athletics.

I also understand that the NCAA, Conference, media, and professional teams may not be covered by the Buckley Amendment or HIPAA and that these regulations may not apply to their use or disclosure of my injury/illness information.

This authorization/consent expires 380 days from the date of my signature below, but I have the right to revoke it in writing at any time by sending written notification to the athletic director at my institution. I understand that a revocation is not effective to the extent action has already been taken in reliance on this authorization/consent.

Printed Name of Student Athlete   Signature   Date

If under age 18:

Signature of Parent or Guardian (identify which)   Date

C.   Shared Responsibility for Sport Safety

Participation in sport requires an acceptance of risk of injury. Athletes rightfully assume that those who are responsible for the conduce of sport have taken reasonable precaution to minimize such risk and that their peers participating in the sport will not intentionally inflict injury upon them.

Periodic analysis of injury patterns and refinements in the rules and other safety decisions in an ongoing process. However to legislate safety via a rule book and equipment

(Continued...)

standards, while often necessary, seldom is effective by itself; and to rely on officials to enforce compliance with the rule book is an insufficient as to rely on warning labels to produce compliance with safety guidelines. "Compliance" means respect on everyone's part for the intent and purpose of a rule or guideline.

I understand that by voluntarily participating in athletics at collegiate level, I am undertaking a non-controllable risk which may result in an injury that may be very severe in nature. Such an injury may result in paralysis and/or death. It is further my understanding that it is entirely my responsibility to report any illness or injury to the athletic training staff or team physician(s). If I do not the University of Nevada will not be responsible for those injuries. A student participating in intercollegiate athletics who reports to a physician without the knowledge of the certified athletic trainer in charge will accept the personal responsibility and expenses of such action. Exceptions are made for away games and during the absence of the athletic trainer at the time of the accident/emergency. I also understand that I must refrain from practice or play while ill or injured. The full-time athletic training staff, through the direction of the team physician(s) will inform the athlete and respective coaching staff of all athlete's injuries and playing/practicing status.

The University of Nevada does not require that all students enroll in the Student Health Service Plan. The University of Nevada Athletic Program expects the student-athletes to obtain Basic Health Care coverage through the Student Health Center at the time of registration. Illness and injuries not directly associated with athletic participation are the responsibility of the student athlete. The University of Nevada insurance policy provides insurance for injuries sustained while participating in play or practice and is "EXCESS COVERAGE ONLY". This means that it pays benefits only after taking into consideration the insurance plan held by you or your parent(s).

I understand sickness and/or injuries are common in all athletics and that the University of Nevada Intercollegiate Athletic Department will provide the most reasonable medical coverage in order to reduce the severity of such illness and/or injuries. The administration, coaches, athletic trainer, and managers will equally provide to each student, equipment required to produce the safest possible intercollegiate athletic environment regardless of age, sex, race, or religion.

I understand that the athletic medical insurance does not cover me until I have been cleared by an athletic medical physical examination. I further understand that the University of Nevada athletic medical insurance if for coverage of athletic injuries/illnesses not directly related to participation in intercollegiate athletics.

I have read the following (pertains to football only)

> **WARNING:** Do not use this helmet to butt, ram or spear opposing players. This is a violation of the football rules and can result in severe head, brain or neck injury, paralysis, or death to you and possible injury to your opponent. There is a risk to you and possible injury to

(Continued...)

Konin JG, Frederick MA. *Documentation for Athletic Training*. Thorofare, NJ: SLACK Incorporated; 2005.

your opponent. There is a risk that injuries may occur as a result of accidental contact without intent to butt, ram or spear. NO HELMET CAN PREVENT ALL SUCH INJURIES. (This information can be found inside every helmet and should be read daily.)

I have been instructed on and issued all necessary equipment that is standard of the NCAA rules.

I have read the above shared responsibility statement and understand that there are certain inherent risks involved in participating in intercollegiate athletics. I acknowledge the fact that these risks exist and I am willing to assume responsibility for such risks while participating at the University of Nevada.

Date:_____   _____
                                                          Signature

Signature may be that of athlete over   _____
18 years of age: if under 18, please   Social Security Number
have parent or guardian sign.

                                                          _____
                                                          Parent or Guardian

D.   AIDS AND INTERCOLLEGIATE ATHLETICS

The Acquired Immunodeficiency Syndrome (AIDS) is caused by a virus or HIV (Human Immunodeficiency Virus). HIV has been isolated in blood, semen, vaginal secretions, saliva, tears, breast milk, cerebrospinal fluid, amniotic fluid, and urine. However, available evidence has implicated only blood, semen, vaginal secretion, and possibly breast milk in the transmission of HIV.

The risk of infection is increased by having multiple sex partners, unprotected sex, and in sharing needles among intravenous drug users.

Although the precise risks of transmission during exposure of open wounds or mucous membrane contaminated blood is not known, theoretically there is a possibility of HIV transmission by blood from one student-athlete to an open wound of another student-athlete.

Therefore, the intercollegiate athletic department, team precautions as recommended by the Center of Disease Control in care of all student-athletes, since medical history and examination cannot reliably verify HIV infected patients.

In addition the Student Health Center on campus will provide HIV testing (fee required) to all students who so request. Information on testing dates may be obtained in the University of Nevada Sports Medicine Center for athletes or by calling the Student Health Center at 784-6598.

(Continued...)

Date:_____

_____
Signature

Signature may be that of athlete over
18 years of age: if under 18, please
have parent or guardian sign.

_____
Social Security Number

_____
Parent or Guardian

Konin JG, Frederick MA. *Documentation for Athletic Training*. Thorofare, NJ: SLACK Incorporated; 2005.

Student Athlete Authorization/Consent
for
Disclosure of Protected Health Information
to the
(name of conference/media outlet, etc.)

I, _____, hereby authorize _____
       Name of Student Athlete   Name of My Institution

and its physicians, athletic trainers and health care personnel to disclose my protected health information and any related information regarding any injury or illness during my training for and participation in intercollegiate athletics to the (name of conference/media outlet, etc.) and its employees or agents.

I understand that my protected health information will be used by the (name of conference/media outlet, etc.) for the purpose of (list purposes).

I understand that my injury/illness information is protected by federal regulations under either the Health Information Portability and Accountability Act (HIPAA) or the Family Educational Rights and Privacy Act of 1974 (the Buckley Amendment) and may not be disclosed without either my authorization under HIPAA or my consent under the Buckley Amendment. I understand that my signing of this authorization/consent is voluntary and that my institution will not condition any health care treatment or payment, enrollment in a health plan or receipt of any benefits (if applicable) on whether I provide the consent or authorization requested for this disclosure. I also understand that I am not required to sign this authorization/consent in order to be eligible for participation in NCAA or conference athletics.

I also understand that the (name of conference/media outlet) is not covered by the Buckley Amendment or HIPAA and that these regulations will not apply to the (conference/media outlet)'s use or disclosure of my injury/illness information.

This authorization/consent expires 380 days from the date of my signature below, but I have the right to revoke it in writing at any time by sending written notification to the athletic director at my institution. I understand that a revocation is not effective to the extent action has already been taken in reliance on this authorization/consent.

_____
Printed Name of Student Athlete   Signature   Date

Konin JG, Frederick MA. *Documentation for Athletic Training*. Thorofare, NJ: SLACK Incorporated; 2005.

SMS - Intercollegiate Athletics-Pre-Participation Examination & Clearance

MHQ _____ INS. INF. _____ INS. Card _____ HIPAA REL _____ PPE Date _____

Athlete: _____ Spt: _____ Date of birth: _____

Height: _____ Weight: _____ Pulse: _____ BP _____ / _____ (_____ / _____ , _____ / _____)

Vision R 20/ _____ L 20/ _____ Corrected: Y N   Pupils: Equal _____ Unequal _____

	NORMAL	ABNORMAL FINDINGS	INITIALS
MEDICAL			
Appearance			
Head			
Eyes/Ears/Nose/Throat			
Lymph Nodes			
Heart		ECHO: EKG:	
Pulses			
Lungs			
Abdomen			
Genitalia (males only)			
Skin			
MUSCULOSKELETAL			
Neck			
Back			
Shoulder/arm			
Elbow/forearm			
Wrist/hand			
Hip/thigh			
Knee			
Leg/ankle			
Foot			

FRESH	SOPH	JUNIOR	SENIOR	FIFTH YR	JR COL./TRANSFER

CLEARANCE

☐ Cleared
☐ Cleared after completing evaluation/rehabilitation for: _____

_____
_____
_____
_____
_____
_____
_____

☐ Not cleared for: _____ Reason: _____

Recommendations: _____
_____
_____

_____ Date: _____
Signature of Physician

Konin FG, Frederick MA. Documentation for Athletic Training. Thorofare, NJ: SLACK Incorporated; 2005.

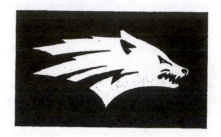

University of Nevada
Intercollegiate Pre-Participation
Physical Examination Form

This form must be complete and on file before the athlete is eligible to participate in Intercollegiate Athletics at the University of Nevada.

Name of Student Athlete _____   Sport _____

Date of Birth _____   SSN _____

Local Address: _____
　　　　　　　　　　Street　　　　　　　　City　　　　State　　　　Zip Code
Local Phone: _____   Cell Phone: _____

Parents/Guardian Name(s) _____

Permanent Address: _____
　　　　　　　　　　　　Street　　　　　　　　City　　　State　　　Zip Code
Parent's Home Phone: _____   Parent's Work Phone: _____

Emergency Contact Name and Phone Number: _____

_____

Eligibility Level: FR SO JR SR   Did you use your redshirt year?   Yes   No

Office Use Only

Ht: _____   Wt: _____   BP: _____/_____   Pulse: _____

KT 1000 score   R _____   L _____

Unconditionally: Cleared: _____   Postponed: _____

Recommendations/Referrals:

_____

_____

_____

Certified Athletic Trainer's Signature: _____   Date: _____

Physician's Signature: _____   Date: _____

Konin JG, Frederick MA. Documentation for Athletic Training. Thorofare, NJ: SLACK Incorporated; 2005.

Physician's Pre-participation Evaluation

MEDICAL	NORMAL	ABNORMAL FINDINGS
Appearance		
Eyes/Ears/Nose/Throat		
Lymph Nodes		
Heart		
Pulses		
Lungs		
Abdomen		
Genitalia (Males only)		
Skin		

Clearance:

☐ Cleared
☐ Cleared after completing evaluation/rehabilitation for:_____

_____
_____
_____
_____
_____

☐ Not Cleared   Reason:_____
Recommendations:_____

_____
_____
_____
_____

Physician's Name (Please print):_____ Date:_____

***Physicians – Please put your signature on front page**

Konin JG, Frederick MA. *Documentation for Athletic Training.* Thorofare, NJ: SLACK Incorporated; 2005.

EXIT MEDICAL ASSESSMENT ACKNOWLEDGEMENT

I have completed my eligibility or am terminating my interest in athletic participation at Southwest Missouri State University and find myself physically

☐   able to function in normal daily activities without
     medical concerns needed to improve my physical status.

☐   am not able to function in normal daily activities and
     have the following concerns about my physical well being.
     (Please provide information below on any and/or all of your
     physical concerns - additional sheets may be attached
     with the information.) If there are concerns, follow-up
     evaluations shall be scheduled through Athletic Training
     Services.

_____   _____
Signature   Date

_____   _____
Print Name   Sport

Konin JG, Frederick MA. *Documentation for Athletic Training*. Thorofare, NJ: SLACK Incorporated; 2005.

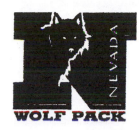

WOLF PACK

UNIVERSITY OF NEVADA
SENIOR CHECKOUT EVALUATION

      The senior checkout evaluation is a post-participation physical exam given to student-athletes whose athletic eligibility at the University of Nevada has ended. The purpose of the exam is to identify any injuries and/or illnesses that the athlete suffered while participating in intercollegiate athletics at the University of Nevada and determine if the athlete will need further medical assistance for those conditions.

      The University of Nevada will assist the student-athlete with medical treatment and payment for injuries and/or illnesses acquired while an active participant in intercollegiate athletics at the University of Nevada for up to ONE (1) YEAR FROM THE DATE OF THE LAST SCHEDULED EVENT OR CONTEST THAT THE STUDENT-ATHLETE PARTICIPATED IN.

      The athlete must report to the training room within two weeks of his or her last scheduled event or contest and receive his or her exam. Failure to do so will result in the athlete being declared clear of all medical conditions and the University of Nevada will no longer be responsible for medical care or payment assistance for the athlete.

Status of Athlete: ☐   Cleared-No existing problem

          ☐   Not Cleared-Existing problems

Notes/Comments: _____

_____

_____

_____

_____

_____

_____

_____

Signature of Athlete: _____ **Date:** _____

Signature of Athletic Trainer: _____ **Date:** _____

UNIVERSITY OF NEVADA
SENIOR CHECKOUT EVALUATION

Name: _____   Sport: _____

Height: _____   Weight: _____   BP: _____/_____   Pulse: _____

Answer the following questions regarding your medical history while participating in intercollegiate athletics at the University of Nevada. If you answer Yes to any of the questions below, please explain the injury/illness, give the dates injured, and list any doctors you may have seen and dates of surgery related to the condition. You may write on the back side of the page if necessary.

1. Have you had any illnesses while participating in intercollegiate athletics at the University of Nevada?

_____No

_____Yes   If Yes, please explain:_____

_____

_____

2. Have you suffered any injuries to your head or neck during your career?

_____No

_____Yes   If Yes, please explain:_____

_____

_____

3. Have you suffered any injuries to either shoulder during your career?

_____No

_____Yes   If Yes, please explain:_____

_____

_____

4. Have you suffered any injuries to your elbow or forearm during your career?

_____No

_____Yes   If Yes, please explain:_____

_____

_____

5. Have you suffered any injuries to your wrists or hands during your career?

_____No

_____Yes   If Yes, please explain:_____

_____

_____

6. Have you suffered any injuries to your cervical, thoracic, or lumbar spine during your career?

_____No

_____Yes   If Yes, please explain:_____

_____

_____

(Continued...)

UNIVERSITY OF NEVADA
SENIOR CHECKOUT EVALUATION

7. Have you suffered any injuries to your hips, pelvis, or upper leg during your career?

_____No

_____Yes   If Yes, please explain:_____

_____

_____

8. Have you suffered any injuries to your knees during your career?

_____No

_____Yes   If Yes, please explain:_____

_____

_____

9. Have you suffered any injuries to your lower legs during your career?

_____No

_____Yes   If Yes, please explain:_____

_____

_____

10. Have you suffered any injuries to your ankles during your career?

_____No

_____Yes   If Yes, please explain:_____

_____

_____

11. Have you suffered any injuries to your feet during your career?

_____No

_____Yes   If Yes, please explain:_____

_____

_____

12. Do you have or have had any medical conditions during your career which were not listed above?

_____No

_____Yes   If Yes, please explain:_____

_____

_____

_____

_____

_____

_____

_____

_____

_____

_____

_____

Name: _____   Sport: _____

Konin JG, Frederick MA. *Documentation for Athletic Training.* Thorofare, NJ: SLACK Incorporated; 2005.

James Madison University - Department of Sports Medicine

Exit Medical Assessment Form

Name: _____

Sport: _____   Exit Year: _____

The following injuries/illnesses are medically documented as having occurred as a direct result of participation in intercollegiate athletic at JMU:

Body Area	Condition	Mo/Yr	Resolved	Unresolved	Findings/Treatment/Status
Head					
Neck					
Shoulder					
Elbow/Forearm					
Wrist/Hand					
Chest					
Abdomen					
Back					
Hip/Groin					
Knee					
Ankle/Foot					

Do you currently have any of the following conditions or illnesses to body systems listed that are unresolved:

☐ Stress Fracture ☐ Concussion ☐ Seizures ☐ Burner/Stinger ☐ Asthma ☐ Diabetes ☐ Ear Infection
☐ Skin Disorder ☐ Nutritional Disorder ☐ Mono ☐ Heart ☐ Allergies ☐ Shin Splints ☐ Depression
☐ Lungs ☐ Compartment Syndrome ☐ Reproductive Organs ☐ Vision ☐ Drug/Alcohol ☐ Teeth
☐ Other _____

(Continued...)

Konin JG, Frederick MA. *Documentation for Athletic Training*. Thorofare, NJ: SLACK Incorporated; 2005.

☐ I have been examined by the JMU Department of Sports Medicine and the above information is accurate. I agree not to hold JMU responsible for any injuries or illnesses that are not aforementioned. I understand that any unresolved conditions may be able to receive financial assistance from JMU on a case-by-case basis if deemed necessary and appropriate by the Director of Sports Medicine and as long as procedures for care as previously outlined by the Department of Sports Medicine in the student athlete handbook have been followed. _____ *(athlete please initial)*

☐ I have been examined by the JMU Department of Sports Medicine and the above information is accurate. I agree not to hold JMU responsible for any injuries or illnesses that are not aforementioned and acknowledge that there are no existing illnesses/injuries that need to be attended to with follow-up care. _____ *(athlete please initial)*

_____ _____
Print Name   Signature   Date

_____ _____
Team Physician   Signature   Date

_____ _____
Supervising ATC   Signature   Date

_____ _____
Director of Sports Medicine   Signature   Date

Konin FG, Frederick MA. Documentation for Athletic Training. Thorofare, NJ: SLACK Incorporated; 2005.

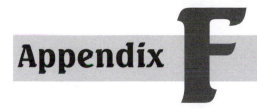

Appendix F

COMMONLY USED FORMS—
PRIVACY FORMS

These forms are designed to inform athletes, patients, and parents/guardians of all the rights and privacy privileges associated with receiving health care services. Forms pertain to insurance coverage and confidentiality policies.

CONTENTS

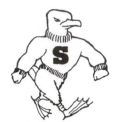

SALISBURY UNIVERSITY

Department of Intercollegiate Athletics, 1101 Camden Avenue
Salisbury, Maryland 21801-6860
www.salisbury.edu/athletics

410-548-3503
FAX 410-546-2639
TTY 410-543-6083

Memo

To: Parents & Guardians of SU athletes

From:

Subject: HMO, PPO, POS, PPN Managed Care Insurance Carriers

I am writing to address a dilemma we are facing at Salisbury University concerning medical coverage for your son or daughter or dependant. If you have an insurance carrier that is an HMO, PPO, POS or PPN Managed Care provider you should be aware of the limitations of your coverage. Most have limited treatment areas or networks, which makes it difficult if not impossible to get elective medical services done while away at school. For instance, if your child injures his or her knee and it appears to be an injury that may require a physician's evaluation, a x-ray or any other elective test, most managed care providers will require the athlete to return home to see the primary care physician. This can delay treatment and become very frustrating for athletes and parents. In addition, there is the burden of traveling back and forth for appointments which may cause the student to miss considerable class time. Though there is no simple solution to this problem I would like to propose some alternatives that you may want to consider to help us combat this problem.

A couple of things to consider. We have a facility that is state of the art for the rehabilitation of athletic injuries, most or all rehabilitation for in season athletes is provided at no cost to your insurance carrier, and with a surgically treated injury this cost alone could be substantial. At least once a week our team orthopedic surgeon visits the athletic training room to evaluate injured athletes. There is no charge for this evaluation, however from this evaluation a treatment plan is formulated. This treatment plan may include x-rays, further testing, recommendation for surgical intervention or any number of treatments which are deemed necessary. This service of having the orthopedist available on a regular basis gives us instant feedback and helps us aggressively move forward in caring for injuries. Another free service is the use of the college student health service. They are at our disposal and are extremely helpful in treating non-orthopedic conditions. What I have tried to outline is the medical services we provide for each student athlete while they are in season. We feel it is comprehensive, experienced and extremely knowledgeable in regards to caring for athletes.

Our problems stem from the inability to render further treatment plans after our physician's initial evaluation. Often times, managed care providers will not permit the next step in care unless the primary care physician is seen. If you are from Baltimore or New York or from parts unknown, this means leaving campus, missing school time and arranging schedules to have an injury evaluated and treated. Often care may be delayed by days and many times weeks.

To help bridge the gap I have some suggestions which will allow us some flexibility in treating your child if they do get injured.

    #1   Change your child's primary care provider to a local physician in Salisbury
    #2   Ask your insurance company about a rider for out of network services for students
    #3   Contact your primary care physician and get pre-approval for any injuries incurred while at school
    #4   Consider another insurance carrier, some may be more expensive however coverage is more comprehensive

It should be noted, most managed care providers do not provide the information I have outlined. You may need to ruffle some feathers, however in the long run I feel we can save time and money in getting your child the proper care. Thank you and please contact me should you have any questions regarding this matter.

1

Konin JG, Frederick MA. *Documentation for Athletic Training*. Thorofare, NJ: SLACK Incorporated; 2005.

SALISBURY UNIVERSITY INSURANCE INFORMATION

The Athletics Department carries an **Excess Insurance** policy that covers each student athlete participating in or traveling to or from an organized practice or game. The policy carries a $1,000 deductible. Therefore, the Athletics Department depends on your personal insurance to absorb this deductible. Every effort will be made to contact you concerning any injuries that may require making an insurance claim. At no time should you pay any bills without consulting the head athletic trainer or our insurance company. If you pay any bill without contacting the athletic trainer or insurance company, reimbursement is highly unlikely.

If the student athlete has no personal health insurance, the Athletics Department will meet the $1,000 deductible. If our insurance carrier deems the claim non-payable, SU Athletics will pay up to the amount of the maximal allowed deductible and nothing more. All claims must originate from the athletic trainer. All referrals to physicians will be made in cooperation with the athletic trainer. **Any referrals made without the prior knowledge of the athletic trainer will not be the responsibility of the SU Athletics Department. Any questions should be referred to the athletic trainer.**

It is extremely important the insurance information on the proceeding page be accurate and complete. It is especially critical to give all necessary claim information if a Health Maintenance Organization (H.M.O.) or Preferred Provider Organization/Network (PPO/PPN) insures you. We will make every attempt to contact these providers prior to seeking out of network or out of area medical attention, **however**, you are ultimately responsible for contacting them and getting permission to treat out of network or out of area should that need arise. We will work very closely with you and your insurance provider to insure proper coverage and payment. If there is a physician within your HMO or PPO/PPN network who is in the Salisbury region you may want to switch your child's care to this physician. This would aid in getting prompt care without the student athlete leaving the Salisbury area.

One last note: The parent, guardian or spouse form must be completed by the next of kin even if the student athlete is not a dependent. **No student athlete will be permitted to practice or play without this form completed by the next of kin.**

Konin JG, Frederick MA. *Documentation for Athletic Training.* Thorofare, NJ: SLACK Incorporated; 2005.

PARENT OR SELF/ INSURANCE INFORMATION FORM

ATHLETE /PARENT/GUARDIAN TO
COMPLETE AND RETURN TO: SOUTHWEST MISSOURI STATE UNIVERSITY

FAILURE TO COMPLETE ALL BLANKS WILL RESULT IN CLAIMS PROCESSING DELAYS.
NOTE: Complete all blanks. If information is not applicable, indicate the reason: e.g., deceased, divorced, unknown.

1. Name: _____ Social Security No: _____
   Sport: _____ Athlete's Birthdate: _____

   Permanent Home Address: _____
   City/State/ZipCode: _____
   Home Phone: _____

2. Father/Guardian: _____ Mother/Guardian: _____
   Birthdate: _____ Birthdate: _____
   Social Security #: _____ Social Security #: _____

   Address: _____ Address: _____

   _____ _____

   Telephone: _____ Telephone: _____

3. Father's Employer: _____ Mother's Employer: _____

   Address: _____ Address: _____

   _____ _____

   Telephone: _____ Telephone: _____

   DO YOU HAVE GROUP MEDICAL INSURANCE COVERAGE ON YOUR SON/DAUGHTER
   THROUGH YOUR EMPLOYER?   Circle: YES   NO

4. **Primary Insurance coverage under:** (circle one) 5. **Secondary Insurance coverage under:** (circle one)
   Father, Mother, Guardian, Athlete, None   Father, Mother, Guardian, Athlete, None

6. **Ins. Company:** _____ **Ins. Company:** _____
   Address: _____ Address: _____

   _____ _____

   _____ _____

   Policy #: _____ Policy #: _____
   Group #: _____ Group #: _____

   Telephone: _____ Telephone: _____

   Primary Care Physician: _____

   PCP Phone #: _____

PLEASE ENCLOSE A <u>COPY OF THE FRONT AND BACK OF YOUR</u> <u>INSURANCE CARD.</u> THANK YOU.

OVER-PLEASE COMPLETE OTHER SIDE ⟹

(Continued...)

Konin JG, Frederick MA. *Documentation for Athletic Training.* Thorofare, NJ: SLACK Incorporated; 2005.

I/We hereby authorize Southwest Missouri State University (Southwest Missouri State University) and the insurance company, or its representatives to inspect or secure copies of case history records, laboratory reports, diagnoses, x-rays, and any other data covering this and/or previous confinements and/or disabilities. A Photostat copy of this authorization shall be deemed as effective and valid as the original.

I/We authorize that Southwest Missouri State University's insurance agent pay directly to Southwest Missouri State University who will pay the medical vendors for any bills incurred from accidents that are covered under the insurance coverage purchased by Southwest Missouri State University.

I/We agree that what ever falls outside Southwest Missouri State University policy for coverage I assume responsibility for.

I/WE AGREE THAT ALL INFORMATION PROVIDED IN THIS DOCUMENT IS ACCURATE AND COMPLETE TO THE BEST OF MY/OUR KNOWLEDGE. I/WE UNDERSTAND THAT ANY INCORRECT OR UNDISCLOSED INFORMATION CANRESULT IN DUPLICATE PAYMENTS CREATINGA SUBSTANTIAL OVERPAYMENT. THE RESPONSIBILITY OF SUCH OCERPAYMENT WILL BE THE OBLIGATION OF THE UNDERSIGNED TO REIMBURSE IN FULL, UPON RERQUEST, ALL AMOUNTS DEEMED REFUNDABLE.

ALL APPROPRIATE SIGNATURES ARE NECESSARY.

PARENT/GUARDIAN/FATHER _____ DATE_____

PARENT/GUARDIAN/MOTHER _____ DATE_____

STUDENT / ATHLETE _____ DATE_____

I DO NOT HAVE ANY MEDICAL INSURANCE COVERAGE ON MY SON/DAUGHTER.
(Only sign if you do **NOT**)

PARENT/ GUARDIAN/FATHER _____ DATE_____

PARENT/GUARDIAN/MOTHER _____ DATE_____

- -

I DO NOT HAVE MEDICAL INSURANCE COVERAGE.

STUDENT/ATHLETE _____ DATE _____

Parent Information Form

Athlete's Name (Print) _____   Social Security # _____

Date of Birth _____   Sport _____   Date _____

SU Athletics Department Insurance Policy Statement:

The Athletics Department provides athletic injury insurance for all varsity athletes for injuries sustained during any organized SU athletic practice or competition, including in-season and out-of-season practices. This policy is "**EXCESS**" or "**SECONDARY**" to any collectible insurance coverage provided by the parents, guardians or self. In the event of any injury occurring as part of an organized SU athletics practice or competition which requires billable medical coverage, a claim will be made to your insurance provider. SU's Athletics Department will not pay on any claim until your insurance has acted on the claim. Please refer to the **INSURANCE INFORMATION BOOKLET** for a more detailed explanation. In addition, if any injury occurs, a detailed billing explanation letter will be sent to you.

THE ATHLETICS DEPARTMENT HIGHLY RECOMMENDS YOU HAVE SOME TYPE OF ACCIDENT INSURANCE COVERAGE WHILE PARTICIPATING IN INTERCOLLEGIATE ATHLETICS.

PLEASE PROVIDE THE INFORMATION REQUESTED BELOW. THIS INFORMATION IS CRITICAL TO PROMPT TREATMENT AND ACCURATE BILLING PROCEDURE. AN INCOMPLETE FORM WILL DELAY THE PARTICIPATION OF THE ATHLETE.

I hereby authorize Salisbury University and their athletic insurance provider, to inspect and secure copies of case history records, laboratory reports, diagnoses, x-rays and any other pertinent data records to previous injuries and/or disabilities. A photo static copy of this authorization shall be deemed as effective and valid as the original.

We/I authorize Salisbury University and their athletic insurance provider to pay medical vendors direct for any bills incurred from accidents' injuries that are covered under the coverage purchased by Salisbury University.

Parent/Guardian Signature: _____	Parent/Guardian Signature: _____
Father/Guardian: _____	Mother/Guardian: _____
Father Social Security: _____	Mother Social Security: _____
Address: _____	Address: _____
Home Telephone: _____	Home Telephone: _____
Employer: _____	Employer: _____
Address: _____	Address: _____
Work Telephone: _____	Work Telephone: _____

Medical Insurance Information (left & right)
Company/Plan, Address, Policy #, Group #, Telephone #, HMO, PPO

Pre-Authorization for Services ☐ Yes ☐ No
Primary Care Physician / Address / Telephone (both columns)

Is a second opinion required before surgery? ☐Yes ☐No
My son/daughter is covered by my own personal insurance ☐Yes ☐No
My son/daughter has their own personal insurance. ☐Yes ☐No

Konin JG, Frederick MA. *Documentation for Athletic Training*. Thorofare, NJ: SLACK Incorporated; 2005.

JonesUniversity's Department of Intercollegiate Athletics
Athlete's Insurance Information
(Please Print)

Athlete' Name_____

Parent's Name (Policy Holder)_____

Policy Holder's Social Security Number_____

Name and Address of Insurance Company_____

_____

Phone Number of Insurance Company(___)_____

Employer Name and Address_____

Policy Number_____ Group Number_____

Any other Identification_____

Is your policy an HMO?   _____YES _____NO

Primary Care Physician Name and Address_____

_____

Phone Number(___)_____

Has your son/daughter seen the Primary Care Physician in the last 12 months___YES___NO

Is your Policy a PPO?   ___YES ___NO

Does your policy have a deductible   ___YES ___NO

If yes, please list amount of deductible $_____

Does your policy have any medication benefits   ___YES ___NO

If yes, please list provider pharmacies_____

_____

Does your son/daughter have a benefits card   ___YES ___NO

If there are any necessary forms or if it requires any procedures, please list or attach:

_____

Parent /Guardian Signature: _____ Date:_____

If you have <u>NO</u> health insurance, Please see back of Page

(Continued...)

NO INSURANCE CLAUSE

Athlete's Name: _____

I have **NO** health insurance in effect to cover my son/daughter. **I understand that I will be responsible for any accidents, illness, or injuries not related to my son/daughter's participation in conditioning sessions, weight training, practice sessions or actual athletic contest.**

The Department or Intercollegiate Athletics can only pay for those injuries caused by participation in conditioning sessions, weight training, practices or actual games. The selection or physicians for medical treatment will be those that work with the department of Intercollegiate Athletics.

Konin JG, Frederick MA. *Documentation for Athletic Training*. Thorofare, NJ: SLACK Incorporated; 2005.

Understanding of Payment

It is our philosophy that all student athletes at James Madison University receive the best possible healthcare services that we can provide. The ability for the Department of Sports Medicine to achieve such a goal requires communication, collaboration and cooperation between our staff, our student athletes, and the parents of our student athletes.

The Department of Sports Medicine at James Madison University employs and/or contracts with certified athletic trainers, physical therapists, strength and conditioning coaches, general medical practitioners, and specialty medical practitioners. These individuals are ultimately responsible for the care of our student athletes. Student athletes who receive care on the premises of JMU do so as a courtesy of the University.

Anytime a student athlete sees an off-campus healthcare provider at the request and approval of the JMU Department of Sports Medicine, the University will assist in the payment of any medical bills that may be acquired. Under these circumstances, the student athlete is required to file the claim under his/her primary insurance carrier and is responsible for all co-payments at the time of rendered service. Once the primary insurance carrier has informed the carrier and medical provider of the amount covered, the student athlete may submit such documents to the Department of Sports Medicine for verification of services provided and payments completed. Once this is done, JMU will allow the medical provider to then file the remainder of the claim under JMU's secondary athletic health care insurance. Any remaining costs incurred by the student athlete following the filing of both primary and secondary insurance should be reported to the JMU Department of Sports Medicine with appropriate documentation. When a student athlete does not have a primary insurance carrier, or when proof of denial for payments by a primary insurance carrier is documented, JMU will again assist the student athlete through the secondary insurance policy.

The Department of Sports Medicine at JMU is not responsible for any medical or healthcare related bills acquired by a student athlete when a student athlete is assessed, evaluated, treated, or consulted with by any provider without the knowledge and written pre-authorization of the Department of Sports Medicine.

By signing below, I acknowledge that I have read and fully understand the guidelines for payment of medical and healthcare related expenses at James Madison University.

_____	_____
Student Athlete Name	Parent Name
_____	_____
Student Athlete Signature	Parent Signature
_____	_____
Date	Date

Konin JG, Frederick MA. *Documentation for Athletic Training*. Thorofare, NJ: SLACK Incorporated; 2005.

JEFF's HIGH SCHOOL
Athletic Insurance Selection Form

Jeff's School Board, its employees, agents, and insurers have no liability, and accepts no liability for injuries or accidents occurring to students during their participation in interscholastic athletics or sports and related extra-curricular teams or activities. The student and parent(s)/guardian(s) assume any and all risks, including without limitation risk of incurring medical expenses associated with the participation by the student.

Student's Name_____ Grade_____
　　　(Print)

_____ We have received an insurance packet from a Jeff's School Board employee, and do not wish to purchase any such insurance, and do hereby affirm our agreement to be responsible for providing insurance covering injuries to the undersigned student athlete.

_____ We have received an insurance packet from a Jeff's School Board employee, and have purchased said insurance, and proof of said purchase is attached.

Parent's Signature_____Date_____

Student's Signature _____ Date_____
　　　(If over age 18)

Konin JG, Frederick MA. *Documentation for Athletic Training.* Thorofare, NJ: SLACK Incorporated; 2005.

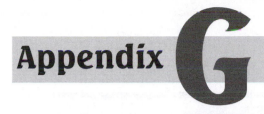

Appendix G

COMMONLY USED FORMS—
RELEASE FORMS

These forms serve to allow patients to formally be informed and acknowledge any sharing of personal medical information with additional parties. Information may include, but is not limited to, health status and insurance records. These forms also educate athletes and patients of safety risks associated with participation in a given sport, activity, or usage of certain equipment.

CONTENTS

All forms reprinted with permission from original source.

Department of Sports Medicine

Medical Information Release Form

Requesting Party

Name: _____   Organization: _____

Phone: _____   Email: _____

Fax: _____   Date of Request: _____

Mailing Address: _____
                                   _____
                                   _____

Student Athlete's Name: _____   Sport: _____

Specific Information Requested: _____

Reason for Request: _____
                               _____
                               _____

I, _____ (print name), do hereby request the aforementioned and agree to use such information solely for the purposes requested.

_____   _____
     Signature   Date

Student Athlete

I, _____ (print name) grant permission for the James Madison University Department of Sports Medicine to provide the requested medical information to the signed party noted above.

_____   _____
     Signature   Date

Processed By: _____   Date: _____   ☐ Fax   ☐ Mail

Please complete and fax this form to (540) 568-

Konin JG, Frederick MA. *Documentation for Athletic Training*. Thorofare, NJ: SLACK Incorporated; 2005.

Jones University

ATHLETIC DEPARTMENT

<u>RELEASE</u>

WHEREBY, I, THE UNDERSIGNED, AM ABOUT TO PARTICIPATE IN A TRY-OUT FOR AN ATHLETIC TEAM UNDER THE SUPERVISION OF THE JONES UNIVERSITY, A STATE OF LOUISIANA INSTITUTION;

WHEREAS, I AM DOING SO ENTIRELY UPON MY OWN INITIATIVE (WITHOUT ANY INCENTIVE OR BEING COERCED), RISK, AND RESPONSIBILITY;

NOW, THEREFORE, IN CONSIDERATION OF THE PERMISSION EXTENDED TO ME TO PARTICIPATE IN THE JONES UNIVERSITY TRY-OUT, I DO HEREBY FOR MYSELF, MY HEIRS, EXECUTORS AND ADMINISTRATORS, REMISE, RELEASE AND FOREVER DISCHARGE AND HOLD HARMLESS JONES UNIVERSITY, ITS COACHES AND ADMINISTRATORS FROM ANY AND ALL CLAIMS, DEMANDS, ACTIONS OR CAUSES OF ACTION ON ACCOUNT OF ANY INJURY TO ME OR ON ACCOUNT OF MY DEATH WHICH MAY OCCUR FROM ANY CAUSE DURING SAID TRY-OUT.

THE ABOVE STATEMENTS APPLY TO THE FOLLOWING:

_____

_____

_____
CANDIDATE SIGNATURE

_____
DATE

_____
SPORT

Konin JG, Frederick MA. *Documentation for Athletic Training.* Thorofare, NJ: SLACK Incorporated; 2005.

Confidentiality Agreement

Confidentiality is a cornerstone of building a strong clinical relationship. As an individual who provides health care you may have access to client's/patient's confidential information that includes biographical data, financial information, medical history and other information. You are expected to protect client confidentiality, privacy and security and to follow these and all associated agency guidelines.

You will use confidential information only as needed to perform duties as a member of the faculty or as a registered student in the athletic training education program. This means, among other things, that:

- You will only access confidential information for which you have a need to know.
- You will respect the confidentiality of any verbal communication or reports printed from any information system containing client's/patient's information and handle, store and dispose of these reports appropriately at the University and associated clinical agency.
- You will not in any way divulge, copy, release, loan, alter, or destroy any confidential information except as properly authorized within the scope of all your professional activities.
- You will carefully protect all confidential information. You will take every precaution so that clients/patients, their families, or other persons do not overhear conversations concerning client/patient care or have the opportunity to view client/patient records.
- You will comply with all policies and procedures and other rules of the University and associated agencies relating to confidentiality of information and access codes.
- You understand that the information accessed through all clinical information systems agencies contains sensitive and confidential client/patient care, business, financial and hospital employee information that should only be disclosed to those authorized to receive it.
- You will not knowingly include or cause to be included in any record or report of false, inaccurate or misleading entry.

You understand that violation of this Confidentiality Agreement may result in disciplinary and legal action with fines. By signing this, you agree that you have read, understand and will comply with the Agreement.

Print Name: _____   **Date:**_____

Signature: _____   **Date:** _____

Witness: _____   **Date:** _____

Konin JG, Frederick MA. *Documentation for Athletic Training*. Thorofare, NJ: SLACK Incorporated; 2005.

Clarion Sports Medicine

HELMET RELEASE FORM

As an athlete, you are entitled to know that your helmet is a piece of equipment which must be used in a proper manner. You must understand that the helmet is a protective device and not a weapon.

Do not strike an opponent with any part of this helmet or face mask. This is a violation of football rules and may cause you to suffer severe brain or neck injury, including paralysis or death. Severe brain or neck injury may also occur accidentally while playing football. No helmet can prevent all such injuries. Use **this helmet at your own risk.**

ATHLETE'S RESPONSIBILITY

Along with regular daily use of this helmet, you are also responsible for daily maintenance checks. These daily maintenance checks will help you to ensure the safety of your helmet and provide you with the best protection for you.

1. Upon daily inspection of your helmet, if you notice any parts loose or missing, you are responsible for reporting it to the head coach or athletic trainer immediately.

2. You must wear a mouth piece and chin strap-at all times while using this helmet.

I have read and understand all instructions for the use of a football helmet.

_____   _____
Athlete's Name   Athlete's Signature

_____   _____
Parent or Guardian Signature   Parent or Guardian Signature

Konin JG, Frederick MA. *Documentation for Athletic Training*. Thorofare, NJ: SLACK Incorporated; 2005.

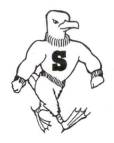

SALISBURY UNIVERSITY

410-548-3503

Department of Intercollegiate Athletics, 1101 Camden Avenue
Salisbury, Maryland 21801-6860
www.salisbury.edu/athletics

FAX 410-546-2639
TTY 410-543-6083

LACROSSE HELMET WARNING STATEMENT

Below is a reprint of the <u>WARNING STATEMENT</u> which is attached to all lacrosse helmets. Please read the statement carefully, it will also be read to you, then sign where indicated to signify that you have read the statement and understand what it implies. If you do not understand the statement contact the Head Athletic Trainer and it will be further explained to you.

<u>WARNING</u>: Lacrosse is a contact sport played with sticks and a hard ball moving at a high speed. This means you can be injured while playing the sport. To reduce the risk of injury, you must exercise common sense and obey the rules at all times. For example, do not use this helmet to butt, ram, or spear another player. This can severely injure you.

Even when you play lacrosse according to the rules you expose yourself to serious injury. <u>THIS HELMET WILL NOT PROTECT YOU AGAINST ALL INJURIES, AMONG OTHERS, NECK AND HEAD INJURIES</u>.

Alteration of this helmet can increase your chances of injury. This helmet should not be worn if cracked or otherwise damaged. Use this helmet for <u>FIELD LACROSSE ONLY</u>.

NAME (print): _____

SIGNATURE: _____

DATE: _____

PARENT, SPOUSE, OR LEGAL GUARDIAN SIGNATURE IF UNDER THE AGE OF 18:

_____

Konin JG, Frederick MA. *Documentation for Athletic Training.* Thorofare, NJ: SLACK Incorporated; 2005.

HELMET WARNING STATEMENT

Below is a reprint of the Warning Statement, which is attached to all football helmets. Please read the statement carefully, and then sign where indicated to signify that you have red the statement and understand what it implies. If you do not understand the statement contact the Head Athletic Trainer and it will be further explained to you.

Do not strike an opponent with any part of this helmet or facemask. This is a violation of football rules and may cause you to suffer severe brain or neck injury, including paralysis or death.
Severe brain or neck injury may also occur accidentally while playing football.

NO HELMET CAN PREVENT ALL SUCH INJURIES.
YOU USE THIS HELMET AT YOUR OWN RISK.

NAME (print): _____

SIGNATURE: _____

DATE: _____

PARENT, SPOUSE, OR LEGAL GUARDIAN SIGNATURE IF UNDER THE AGE OF 18:

_____

Konin JG, Frederick MA. *Documentation for Athletic Training*. Thorofare, NJ: SLACK Incorporated; 2005.

Clarion Sports Medicine

ACKNOWLEDGEMENT OF RISK
AND CONSENT TO PARTICIPATE

I/We hereby acknowledge an awareness that participation in interscholastic athletics involves a risk of injury, which may include severe injuries possibly involving paralysis, permanent mental disability, or death, and that these injuries may occur in some instances as the result of unavoidable accidents. Clarion Area School District has taken appropriate steps to reduce this risk by teaching proper technique, employing a certified athletic trainer and retaining the services of a team physician and EMS personnel as indicated by the assessment of risk. Parents further acknowledge that the Certified Athletic Trainer may contact the student's physician in order to obtain information concerning the extent of injuries sustained, the extent to which a student may participate in the sport, and what additional treatment the physician may want the ATC to perform. Information obtained by the ATC will be considered confidential and will be treated as such. We accept these risks in giving consent to participate in interscholastic athletics.

_____   _____
Print Athlete's Full Name   Athlete's Signature

_____   _____
Print Name of Father or Guardian   Signature of Father or Guardian

_____   _____
Print Name of Mother or Guardian   Signature of Mother or Guardian

Konin JG, Frederick MA. *Documentation for Athletic Training*. Thorofare, NJ: SLACK Incorporated; 2005.

University of Nevada
Department of Intercollegiate Athletics
Awareness of Risk

Name:_____   Sport:_____

      I am aware that playing or practicing in any sport can be a dangerous activity involving many risks or injury. I understand that the dangers and risks of playing or practicing in the above sport(s) include, but are not limited to, death, serious neck and spinal injuries which may result in complete or partial paralysis or brain damage, serious injury to virtually all bones, joints, ligaments, muscles, tendons and other aspects of my body, general health and well being. I furthermore specifically acknowledge that participation in intercollegiate athletics may involve a risk of injury.

      In consideration of UN permitting me to practice, play, try out for or otherwise associate myself with the UN intercollegiate athletics program, and to engage in all activities related to the program, including practicing, playing and travel, I hereby voluntarily assume all risks associated with participation and agree to discharge and release the state of Nevada, the Regents of the University of Nevada, their agents and servants and employees, from any and all liability, claims, causes of action or demands of any kind and nature whatsoever which may arise by or in connection with my participation in any activities related to the intercollegiate athletics program, except where such claims are due to the sole negligence of the University of Nevada, its agents or employees. Because of the inherent dangers of participating in a contact or other type of sport, I recognize the importance of following the coach's instructions regarding playing techniques, training, rules of the sport and other team rules, and agree to obey such instructions.

      The terms hereof shall serve as a release and assumption of risk for my heirs, estate, executor, administrator, assignees, and all members of my family.

<u>Check One of the Following:</u>

☐   I am in good health and I know of no medical reason why I am not able to participate in the University of Nevada intercollegiate athletics program.

☐   I have a significant physical condition that may increase my risk in participating in the University of Nevada intercollegiate athletics program. My specific physical condition(s) is (are): _____ (examples include, but are not limited to, those who have heart disease/conditions, those who have only one functioning organ of a paired organ group, those confined to a wheelchair, those who are deaf, blind or missing a limb, those with severe chronic illness, those with a severe reduction in normal physiologic function, and those who may have a physical, behavioral, emotional, or psychological disorder or abnormality that substantially limits a major life activity). I understand that I will be required to obtain the clearance of the team physician to participate. I further understand that irrespective of the clearance of the team physician, I may be at greater risk of suffering injury, illness, or death as a result of my participation. For the specific additional risks associated with my participation, I understand I should consult with my personal physician and specialist, in addition to the team physician. By continuing to participate in intercollegiate athletics despite these additional risks, I agree to assume these additional risks and waive any claims I may have as set forth more fully in each of the above paragraphs.

I certify that I am at least 18 years of age. If not, parental/guardian signature is required.

Year:_____ Signature:_____ Date:_____

Parent/Guardian Signature (if minor): _____

Date:_____

Konin JG, Frederick MA. *Documentation for Athletic Training*. Thorofare, NJ: SLACK Incorporated; 2005.

Assumption of Risk Statement

I, _____(print name), verify that I have been informed that I may be injured while participating in intercollegiate athletic practice or competition. I understand that it is possible that I may sustain an injury which may result in permanent disability, paralysis, or possibly death. I understand that paralysis may include loss of movement, feeling, and use of my arms, legs, and trunk. I further understand that paralysis may involve complete loss of sexual function, and/or bowel and bladder control, which would require the use of external aids, attached or inserted into my body for the collection and removal of body wastes.

I understand that paralysis and its effects could last my entire lifetime.

In addition, I understand that an injury to any of my body joints may result in disfiguration, loss of movement, strength or feeling which may last my entire lifetime.

I understand that it is my responsibility to adhere to all rules and regulations for my chosen sport. I understand that infraction of the rules may result in injury to myself or my opponent. I also understand that no modification of protective equipment or uniform should be made.

In addition, I understand that it is my responsibility to report faulty or poor-fitting equipment immediately to the coach, equipment manager, or Certified Athletic Trainer.

I understand that all injuries are to be reported to the Certified Athletic Trainer and that I am responsible for the follow-up care and treatment of my injuries under the Certified Athletic Trainer's supervision.

I understand and accept these risks of participation of _____ during the
20 ___ -20___ season.   (Sport)

_____   _____
Student-Athlete Name (Print)   Student-Athlete Signature

_____   _____
Date of Signature   Date of Birth

_____   _____
Parent/Guardian Name if Under 18 (Print)   Parent/Guardian Signature if Under 18

Konin JG, Frederick MA. *Documentation for Athletic Training*. Thorofare, NJ: SLACK Incorporated; 2005.

<u>Clarion Sports Medicine</u>

ATHLETIC TRAINING
CARE/EMERGENCY
AUTHORIZATION

I, _____, hereby give my permission to the NATA Certified Athletic Trainer
       Parent/Guardian print name
employed by Clarion School District to perform immediate care and emergency treatment to injuries
incurred during any interscholastic or intramural activity in this school district, and if necessary, to
transport him/her to the nearest medical facility.

In case of medical emergency, I give my consent to the hospital or
physician to perform or administer emergency care to my son/daughter,_____.
                                                              Athlete's name

_____   Parent/guardian

signature

_____   Parent/guardian

signature

Konin JG, Frederick MA. *Documentation for Athletic Training*. Thorofare, NJ: SLACK Incorporated; 2005.

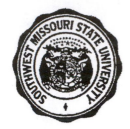

SOUTHWEST MISSOURI STATE UNIVERSITY

Notice of Privacy Practices Acknowledgment Cover Sheet
HIPAA Procedure 1.005, Form 1
Page 1 of 1

Please complete this sheet. This sheet will be filed in your medical record file.

Southwest Missouri State University Health Care Components are required by law to maintain the privacy of protected health information and to provide individuals with notice of its legal duties and privacy practices with respect to Protected Health Information (PHI).

I, _____, student-athlete at SMS, hereby acknowledge that I have received this Notice of Privacy Practices, with an effective date of April 14, 2003.

_____   _____

Student-Athlete's signature or legal guardian signature   Date
of minor child

Notice Effective April 14, 2003

Southwest Missouri State University, Health Care Components (HCC)

Notice of Privacy Practices

Forest Institute Human Services Center
1322 S. Campbell ∽ Springfield, MO 65807
Phone (417) 865-8943 ∽ Fax (417) 831-6839

Consent for Treatment, Financial Agreement, And Patient Bill of Rights
Please Read and Sign at the Bottom of the Page

Patient Name (SMS ATHLETE)	Social Security Number	Date of Birth

Forest Institute Human Services Center is a teaching facility of Forest Institute of Professional Psychology. We provide services to individuals, families, and groups. Services are provided by psychological trainees, interns, and residents supervised by licensed psychologists. Therapy sessions are typically 45 – 50 minutes and scheduled once a week. Depending on your individual circumstances, testing may be ordered to enhance your treatment. Video/Audio taping and observation of therapy and testing sessions are a normal and customary procedure. The taping is for supervisory consultation, training, and research purposes only.

CONFIDENTIALITY

I understand that information related to my treatment is confidential. I further understand that the clinical staff is required by law to release information to appropriate sources in four specific situations:

- There is reasonable belief that I will do harm to myself
- There is reasonable belief that I will do harm to others

- There is reasonable evidence of physical, sexual, or emotional abuse or neglect of a minor or elder
- If subpoenaed by a court of law or court ordered

PATIENT'S BILL OF RIGHTS

- To have all rights of the clinic regardless of race, color, sex, religion, national origin, age or disability
- To have adequate mental health services and treatment in as open a setting as possible
- To have the clinic and its programs explained to him/her clearly and understandably
- To know the name of the person in charge of the treatment and to know approximately how he/she will be under care and to take part in the planning and the discharge
- To have records kept confidential

- To be allowed to meet with his/her attorney and personal physician at will
- To be treated courteously and be free from verbal and physical abuse
- To have charges, billing, insurance and fees explained fully
- To exercise civil rights unless declared legally incompetent
- To have the same legal rights and responsibilities as any other citizen unless otherwise stated by law.

The Forest Human Services Center shall attempt to offer the highest quality Mental Health Services delivered in a professional fashion and atmosphere by trained, competent professionals. Psychological Trainees shall at all times be under the supervision of a licensed professional. The ethical guidelines of the Forest Human Services Center shall be in compliance with the Missouri Psychological Association, State Committee of Psychologists, and the American Psychological Association.

PAYMENT FOR SERVICES

$_____ Individual Therapy for Adult/Child	$_____ Parenting Classes	
$_____ Marital/Couple/Family Therapy	$_____ Group Sessions	
$_____ Assessment	$_____ Other services	

CONSENT FOR TREATMENT

I hereby acknowledge and consent to psychological treatment and/or evaluation for myself, my child or legal ward as deemed appropriate by the clinical staff of Forest Human Services Center. I further understand that my assigned therapist may be a psychological trainee, intern, resident, or assistant who is supervised by a licensed, doctoral level psychologist. I agree to the conditions and rights listed above and agree to pay the designated fee as agreed upon. My intent is to retain psychological services of the Forest Human Services Center.

_____   _____
Signature (Note: Custodial Parent/Guardian must sign for Minor Child)   Date

_____   _____
Witness   Date

Konin JG, Frederick MA. *Documentation for Athletic Training*. Thorofare, NJ: SLACK Incorporated; 2005.

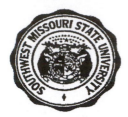

SOUTHWEST MISSOURI STATE UNIVERSITY

Notice of Privacy Practices
HIPAA Procedure 1.005, Form 2
Page 1 of 6

This Notice of Privacy Practices (NPP) describes how health information about you may be used and disclosed and how you can get access to this information. Please review it carefully. If you have any questions about this NPP please contact the University Privacy Officer or a Unit Privacy Officer at one of the University's Health Care Components (HCC).

This NPP will explain:
- How a HCC such as Athletics and Athletic Training Services may use and disclose your Protected Health Information (PHI);
- Our obligations related to the use and disclosure of your PHI;
- Your rights related to any PHI that a HCC has or retains about you.

This NPP describes how a HCC may use and disclose your PHI to carry out treatment, payment and/or health care operations and for other purposes that are permitted or required by law. It also describes your rights to access and control your PHI. PHI is information about you, including demographic information, which may identify you and that relates to your past, present or future physical or mental health or condition and related health care services.

The University HCC are required to abide by the terms of this NPP. A copy is available at all HCCs, and at the below stated website. The University may change the terms of this NPP, at any time. The new NPP will be effective for all PHI that a HCC maintains at that time. The HCC will provide you with any revised NPP by posting it on our website: http://smsu.edu/privacy/hipaa and making it available when you visit a HCC.

I. Uses and Disclosures of Protected Health Information (PHI)

On your first visit to a HCC, you may be asked to complete a new patient information form and you will be required to sign an acknowledgement of NPP. A copy of the NPP will be made available to you. A HCC may obtain, but is not required to, your consent for the use or disclosure of your PHI for treatment, payment and/or health care operations. HCCs are required to obtain your authorization for the use or disclosure of your information for other specific purposes or reasons. HCCs have listed some of the types of uses or disclosures below. Not every possible use or disclosure is covered, but all of the ways that a HCC is allowed to use and disclose information will fall into one of the categories. Your PHI may be used and disclosed by your provider, our office staff and others outside of our office that are involved in your care and treatment for the purpose of providing health care services to you. Your PHI may also be used and disclosed to pay your health care bills and to support the operation of a HCC. Following are examples of the types of uses and disclosures of your PHI that a HCC is permitted to make.

    A.   **Treatment:** A HCC will use and disclose your PHI to provide, coordinate, or manage your health care and any related services. This includes the coordination or management of your PHI with a third party that has already obtained your permission to have access to your PHI. For example, a HCC would disclose your PHI, as necessary, to a home health agency that provides care to you. A HCC will also disclose PHI to other providers or health facilities that may treat you when it has the necessary permission from you to disclose your PHI. For example, your PHI may be provided to a health provider to whom you have been referred to ensure that the provider has the necessary PHI to diagnose or treat you. In addition, a HCC may disclose your PHI from time-to-time to another health care provider (*e.g.*, a specialist or laboratory) who, at the request of your

(Continued...)

Konin JG, Frederick MA. *Documentation for Athletic Training.* Thorofare, NJ: SLACK Incorporated; 2005.

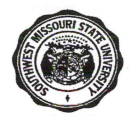

SOUTHWEST MISSOURI STATE UNIVERSITY

Notice of Privacy Practices
HIPAA Procedure 1.005, Form 2
Page 2 of 6

provider, becomes involved in your care by providing assistance with your health care diagnosis or treatment to your provider.

B.   Payment: Your PHI will be used, as needed, to obtain payment for your health care services. This may include certain activities that your health insurance plan may undertake before it approves or pays for the health care services recommended for you such as: making a determination of eligibility or coverage for insurance benefits, reviewing services provided to you for medical necessity, and undertaking utilization review activities. For example, a HCC may need to provide your insurance plan information about treatment you received, so your insurance will pay for the services.

C.   Healthcare Operations: A HCC may use or disclose, as needed, your PHI in order to support the business activities of a HCC. These activities include, but are not limited to: quality assessment activities, licensing, and employee review activities. In addition, a HCC may use a sign-in sheet at the registration desk where you will be asked to sign your name. The staff of a HCC may also call you by name in a lobby when your provider is ready to see you. A HCC may use or disclose your PHI, as necessary, to contact you to remind you of your appointment. A HCC will share your PHI with third party "business associates" that perform various activities (*e.g.*, billing, reading of x-rays, performing lab tests, transcription services) for the practice. Whenever an arrangement between our office and a business associate involves the use or disclosure of your PHI, the HCC will have a written contract that contains terms that will protect the privacy of your PHI.

II.   Uses and Disclosures of Protected Health Information Based upon Your Written Authorization

Other uses and disclosures of your PHI will be made only with your written authorization, unless otherwise permitted or required by law as described below. You may revoke this authorization, at any time, in writing, except to the extent that your provider has taken an action in reliance on the use or disclosure indicated in the authorization.

A.   Research: To comply with laws and regulations other than HIPAA, Taylor Health and Wellness Center, Athletic Training Services, Speech and Hearing Clinic, and other HCCs will not allow your PHI collected by their staff, to be used in research projects without your written consent. Under certain circumstances, the University may use and disclose PHI about you for research purposes when the Institutional Review Board has approved a waiver of authorization for the Protection of Human Subjects. For example, a research project may involve comparing the health and recovery of all patients who received one medication to those who received another for the same condition. All research projects, however, are subject to a special approval process under Missouri law. This process evaluates a proposed research project and its use of health information, trying to balance the research needs with patients' need for privacy of their health information. Before we use or disclose PHI for research, the project will have been approved through this research approval process. The University may, however, disclose PHI about you to people *preparing* to conduct a research project, for example, to help them look for patients with specific medical needs, so long as the health information they review does not leave the facility.

III.   Uses and Disclosures of Protected Health Information That Do Not Require Your Consent or Authorization

(Continued...)

Konin JG, Frederick MA. *Documentation for Athletic Training.* Thorofare, NJ: SLACK Incorporated; 2005.

SOUTHWEST MISSOURI STATE UNIVERSITY

Notice of Privacy Practices
HIPAA Procedure 1.005, Form 2
Page 3 of 6

A HCC can use or disclose PHI about you without your consent or authorization when:
- There is an emergency or when a HCC is required by law to treat you,
- When a HCC is required by law to use or disclose certain information, or
- When there are substantial communication barriers to obtaining consent from you.

A HCC can also use or disclose PHI about you without your consent or authorization for:

A.   Appointment Reminders: A HCC may use and disclose PHI to contact you as a reminder that you have an appointment for treatment or services at a HCC.

B.   Treatment Alternatives and Health-Related Benefits and Services: A HCC may use and disclose PHI to tell you about or recommend possible treatment options or alternatives or health-related benefits or services that may be of interest to you.

C.   Individuals Involved in Disaster Relief: Should a disaster occur, a HCC may disclose PHI about you to any agency assisting in a disaster relief effort so that your family can be notified about your condition, status and location.

D.   As Required By Law: A HCC will disclose PHI about you when required by law.

E.   To Avert a Serious Threat to Health or Safety: A HCC may use and disclose PHI about you when necessary to prevent a serious threat to the health and safety of you, the public, or any other person. However, any such disclosure would only be to someone able to help prevent the threat.

F.   Organ and Tissue Donation: If you are an organ donor, a HCC may release PHI to organizations that handle organ procurement or organ, eye or tissue transplantation or to an organ donation bank, as necessary to facilitate organ or tissue donation and transplantation.

G.   Military and Veterans: If you are a member of the armed forces, a HCC may release PHI about you as required by military command authorities. A HCC may also release PHI about foreign military personnel to the appropriate foreign military authority.

H.   Workers' Compensation: When disclosure is necessary to comply with Workers' Compensation laws or purposes, a HCC may release PHI about you for workers' compensation or similar programs. These programs provide benefits for work-related injuries or illnesses.

I.   Public Health Risks: A HCC may disclose PHI about you for public health activities. These activities generally include the following: to prevent or control disease, injury or disability; to report births and deaths; to report child abuse or neglect; to report reactions to medications or problems with products; to notify people of recalls of products they may be using; to notify a person who may have been exposed to a disease or may be at risk for contracting or spreading a disease or condition or to notify the appropriate government authority if we believe a patient has been the victim of abuse, neglect or domestic violence. The HCC will only make this disclosure if you agree or when required or authorized by law.

J.   Health Oversight Activities: A HCC may disclose PHI to a health oversight agency for activities authorized by law. These oversight activities include, for example, audits, investigations, inspections, and licensure. These activities are necessary for the government to monitor the health care system, government programs, and compliance with civil rights laws.

(Continued...)

Konin JG, Frederick MA. *Documentation for Athletic Training*. Thorofare, NJ: SLACK Incorporated; 2005.

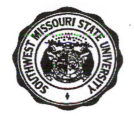

SOUTHWEST MISSOURI STATE UNIVERSITY

Notice of Privacy Practices
HIPAA Procedure 1.005, Form 2
Page 4 of 6

K.   Lawsuits and Disputes: If you are involved in a lawsuit or a dispute, a HCC may disclose PHI about you in response to a court or administrative order as required by law.

L.   Law Enforcement: A HCC may release PHI if asked to do so by a law enforcement official; however, if the material is protected by 42 CFR Part 2 (a federal law protecting the confidentiality of drug and alcohol abuse treatment records), a court order is required. A HCC may also release limited PHI to law enforcement in the following situations: (1) about a patient who may be a victim of a crime if, under certain limited circumstances, the HCC is unable to obtain the patient's agreement; (2) about a death a HCC believes may be the result of criminal conduct; (3) about criminal conduct at the university; (4) about a patient where a patient commits or threatens to commit a crime on the premises or against program staff (in which case the HCC may release the patient's name, address, and last known whereabouts); (5) in emergency circumstances, to report a crime, the location of the crime or victims, and the identity, description and/or location of the person who committed the crime; and (6) when the patient is a forensic client and the HCC is required to share with law enforcement by Missouri statute.

M.   Coroners, Medical Examiners and Funeral Directors: A HCC may release PHI to a coroner or medical examiner. This may be necessary, for example, to identify a deceased person or determine the cause of death. A HCC may also release PHI about patients of the university facilities to funeral directors as necessary to carry out their duties.

N.   National Security and Intelligence Activities: A HCC may release PHI about you to authorized federal officials for intelligence, counterintelligence, and other national security activities authorized by law.

O.   Protective Services for the President and Others: A HCC may disclose PHI about you to authorized federal officials so they may conduct special investigations or provide protection to the President and other authorized persons or foreign heads of state.

P.   Inmates: If you are an inmate of a correctional institution or under the custody of a law enforcement official, PHI may be released about you to the correctional institution or law enforcement official if the release is necessary (1) for the institution to provide you with health care; (2) to protect your health and safety or the health and safety of others; or (3) for the safety and security of the correctional institution.

IV.   Other Uses Or Disclosures Of Protected Health Information

Other uses or disclosures not covered in this NPP will not be made without your written authorization, unless otherwise permitted or required by law. If you provide a HCC with written authorization to use or disclose information, you can change your mind and revoke your authorization at any time, as long as it is in writing. If you revoke your authorization, a HCC will no longer use or disclose the information. However, a HCC will not be able to take back any disclosures that have been made pursuant to your previous authorization.

V.   **Your Rights Regarding Health Information About You**

You have the following rights regarding PHI a HCC maintains about you:

A.   Right to Inspect and Copy: You have the right to inspect and receive a copy of your PHI *with the exception of psychotherapy notes and information compiled in anticipation of litigation.* To inspect and receive a copy of your PHI, you must submit your request in writing to a HCC's Unit Privacy Officer or designee. If you request a

(Continued...)

Konin JG, Frederick MA. *Documentation for Athletic Training*. Thorofare, NJ: SLACK Incorporated; 2005.

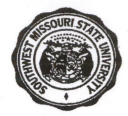

SOUTHWEST MISSOURI STATE UNIVERSITY

Notice of Privacy Practices
HIPAA Procedure 1.005, Form 2
Page 5 of 6

copy of the information, the HCC may charge a fee for the costs of copying, mailing or other supplies associated with your request. A HCC may deny your request to inspect and copy in certain limited circumstances. If you are denied access to your PHI because of a threat or harm issue, you may request that the denial be reviewed. Another licensed health care professional chosen by a HCC will review your request and the denial. The person conducting the review will not be the person who denied your request. The HCC will comply with the outcome of the review.

B.   Right to Request an Amendment: If you feel your PHI that a HCC has about you is incorrect or incomplete, you may ask to have the information amended. You have the right to request an amendment for as long as the information is kept by or for the HCC. Requests for an amendment must be made in writing and submitted to the Unit Privacy Officer or designee. You must provide a reason to support your request for an amendment. A HCC may deny your request if it is not in writing or if it does not include a reason supporting the request. In addition, a HCC may deny your request if you ask us to amend information that:

- Was not created by a HCC, unless the person or entity that created the information is no longer available to make the amendment;
- Is not part of the PHI kept by or for a HCC;
- Is not part of the information which you would be permitted to inspect and copy or;
- Is accurate and complete.

C.   Right to an Accounting of Disclosures: You have the right to request an "accounting of disclosures", a list of the disclosures made by a HCC of your PHI. To request an accounting of disclosures, you must submit your request in writing to the HCC's Unit Privacy Officer or designee. Your request must state a time period which may not go back more than six years and cannot include dates before April 14, 2003. Your request should indicate in what form you want the list (for example, on paper or electronically). The first list you request within a twelve-month period will be free. For additional lists in a twelve-month period, a HCC may charge you for the cost of providing the list. A HCC will notify you what that cost will be and give you an opportunity to withdraw or modify your request before you are charged. There are some disclosures that a HCC does not have to track. For example, when you give a HCC an authorization to disclose some information, the HCC is not required to track that disclosure.

D.   Right to Request Restrictions: You have the right to request a restriction or limitation on the PHI a HCC uses or discloses about you for treatment, payment and/or health care operations. For example, you could ask that a HCC not use or disclose information about your family history to a particular community provider. *The HCC is not required to agree to your request.* If a HCC does agree, it will comply with your request unless the information is needed to provide you emergency treatment. To request restrictions on the use or disclosure of your PHI for treatment, payment or health care operations, you must make your request in writing to the HCC's Unit Privacy Officer or designee. In your request, you must tell a HCC (1) what information you want to limit; (2) whether you want to limit our use, disclosure or both; and (3) to whom you want the limits to apply (for example, disclosures to your spouse).

(Continued...)

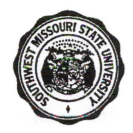

SOUTHWEST MISSOURI STATE UNIVERSITY

Notice of Privacy Practices
HIPAA Procedure 1.005, Form 2
Page 6 of 6

E. **Right to Request Confidential Communications**: You have the right to request that a HCC communicate with you about medical matters in a certain way or at a certain location. For example, you can ask that a HCC only contact you at work or by mail. To request confidential communications, you must make your request in writing to a HCC's Unit Privacy Officer or designee. Your request must specify how or where you wish to be contacted. A HCC will not ask you the reason for your request and will accommodate all reasonable requests.

F. **Right to a Paper Copy of This Notice**: You have the right to a paper copy of this notice even if you have agreed to receive the notice electronically. You may ask a HCC to give you a copy of this notice at any time by contacting the HCC's Unit Privacy Officer or designee. You may also obtain a copy of this notice at our website http://smsu.edu/privacy/hipaa.

VI. Changes To This Notice

The University reserves the right to change this NPP. The University may make the revised notice effective for PHI a HCC already has about you as well as any information a HCC receives in the future. The University will post a copy of the current NPP in all HCCs. The NPP will contain on the first page, in the top right-hand corner, the effective date. In addition, each time you register at or are admitted or apply for services to the HCC for treatment and/or services, you will be offered a copy of the current NPP in effect. If you want to request any revised NPP, you may access it at our website, http://smsu.edu/privacy/hipaa.

VII. Complaints

If you believe your privacy rights have been violated you may:

A. File a complaint with a HCC by contacting its Unit Privacy Officer or Designee by dialing the HCC's main number, or the University's Privacy Officer by dialing the University at (417-836-5000), or by mail: University Privacy Officer, Taylor Health and Wellness Center, Southwest Missouri State University, 901 South National Avenue, Springfield, MO 65804.

B. File a complaint with the University or a HCC or the Secretary of the Department of Health and Human Services. You may call them at 877-696-6775 or write to them at 200 Independence Ave. S.W., Washington, DC, 20201.

C. File a grievance with the Office of Civil Rights by calling 866-OCR-PRIV (866-627-7748), or 886-788-4989 TTY.

All complaints must be submitted in writing. You will not be penalized for filing a complaint.

Effective: April 14, 2003

Konin JG, Frederick MA. *Documentation for Athletic Training.* Thorofare, NJ: SLACK Incorporated; 2005.

TREATMENT AUTHORIZATION: TERMS OF TREATMENT AGREEMENT: HIPAA NOTICE

A. Consent for Treatment: I understand that my outpatient treatment in this facility is indicated because of my condition. I voluntarily authorize and consent to the usual and customary examinations, test, and procedures performed on student-athletes in my condition and the usual and customary care and/or rehabilitation. No guarantees are made by Athletic Training Services Southwest Missouri State University (SMS) as to the results of treatments or examinations. Additionally, among those who provide care to student/athletes and observe it being rendered are health care personnel in training.

B. Authorization To Release Information: I hereby authorize Athletic Training Services (SMS) and my physicians to release any and all information contained in my medical record pertaining to this period of outpatient treatment to: (a) my insurance company and its contractual vendors, (b) third-party carriers and their contractual vendors or their representatives, as necessary for payment of this account, (c) any person or entity participating in the performance of review of the care rendered by Athletic Training Services (SMS) and/or physicians, and also (d) my social security number to the manufacturer of medical devices in accordance with federal law and regulations.

C. Assignment of Benefits: In consideration of the services rendered, I hereby assign any benefits due under my insurance coverage benefits for services to Athletic Training Services (SMS). In the event the above charges are not covered by my insurance, for whatever reason, I will be responsible for payment of the remaining amount not covered by Southwest Missouri State University. I understand the balance of the account is due and payable upon receipt of the statement, unless prior arrangements are made. In the event of a collection, the cost of collection, inclusion of reasonable attorney fees shall be included as part of the obligation due Athletic Training Services (SMS).

D. Acknowledgement: My signature below acknowledges my receipt of information and does not waive any of my rights to request a review or make me liable for any payment. It also, acknowledges that the Health Insurance Portability, and Accountability Act (HIPAA) Notice of Privacy has been made available to me.

The undersigned certifies that the conditions of admission have been read and are understood. The undersigned is the student-athlete or is duly authorized to act on behalf of the student-athlete to execute these conditions of admission and accept the terms thereof.

X_____   _____
SIGNATURE OF ATHLETE / DATE   **WITNESS/DATE**

_____   _____
PRINT NAME LEDGIBLY   **SPORT CODE**

CERTIFICATE MEDICAL NECESSITY/ PHYSICIAN PRESCRIPTION

_____
INJURY/ACCIDENT - ICD CODE

Return to functional daily activities in:_____   _____
                                                                PROGNOSIS   **EST. DURATION OF TX.**

Frequency: **Daily**   **Date Prescribed:**_____

Description of Service: **Care/Rehabilitation of**_____
Prescribing Physician:

                                                                _____
                                                                SIGNATURE

Provider's Name: **Athletic Training Services**
Address: **Southwest Missouri State University**
                         901 South National   _____
                         Springfield, MO 65804   **PROVIDER SIGNATURE**

THIS IS A PERMANENT FILE COPY DO NOT REMOVE

01/20/99-original   04/08/03 revised

Konin JG, Frederick MA. *Documentation for Athletic Training*. Thorofare, NJ: SLACK Incorporated; 2005.

NOTICE OF PRIVACY PRACTICES (effective August 1, 2003)

This notice describes how your health information may be used and disclosed by the University of Nevada Athletic Training Department and your rights pertaining to that information. Please review it carefully.

UNDERSTANDING YOUR PATIENT HEALTH INFORMATION (PHI)

Understanding what is in your health record and how your health information is used will help you to ensure its accuracy, allow you to better understand who, what, where and why others may access your health information, and assist you in making more informed decisions when authorizing disclosure to others. When you visit us, we keep a record of your symptoms, examination, test results, diagnoses, treatment plan, and other medical information. We also may obtain health records from other providers. In using and disclosing your protected health information, it is our objective to follow the Privacy Standards of the federal Health Insurance Portability and Accountability Act, 45 CFR Part 464, even if this is not required in order to treat students. The law allows us to use and disclose your health information without your specific authorization for treatment, payment and operations and other specific purposes explained on the next page. This includes the sharing of information, when necessary and appropriate, with other heath care components of the University, such as the athletic department, student health center or the counseling center, as necessary for your continued care. All other uses and disclosures require your specific authorization.

YOUR HEALTH INFORMATION RIGHTS You have a right to:

- Request a restriction on the uses and disclosures of your protected health information as described in this notice, although we are not required to agree to the restriction you request. You should address your request in writing to the designated Privacy Officer. We will notify you within 30 days if we cannot agree to the restriction.
- If you received the Notice of Privacy Practices electronically, you may request a paper copy of the Notice.
- Upon written request, you may inspect and obtain a copy of your health record for a fee of $.60 per page and the actual cost of postage per **NRS 629.061**, except that you are not entitled to access to, or to obtain a copy of, psychotherapy notes and information compiled for legal proceedings.
- Amend your health record by submitting a written request with the reasons supporting the request to the Privacy Officer. In most cases, we will respond within 30 days. We are not required to agree to the requested amendment.
- Obtain an accounting of disclosures of your health information, except that we are not required to account for disclosures for treatment, payment, operations, or pursuant to authorization, among other exceptions.
- Send and receive confidential communications of protected health information by alternative means or at alternative location, other than our usual methods. You should address the request in writing to the designated Privacy Officer.
- Revoke an authorization to use or disclose health information at any time except where action has already been taken.

RESPONSIBILITIES OF THE UNR ATHLETIC TRAINING DEPARTMENT We are required by law to:

- Maintain the privacy of your protected health information and provide you with notice of our legal duties and privacy practices with respect to your protected health information.
- Abide by the terms of the notice currently in effect. We have the right to change our notice of privacy practices and apply the change to all of your protected health information, including information obtained prior to the change.
- If we change our notice of privacy practices, we will post the new changes in the lobby and a copy will be available to you upon request.
- Use or disclose your health information only with your authorization except as described in this notice.
- In some circumstance, state or federal law may prohibit or further restrict the disclosure of your health information. If that is the case, we are required to follow the more stringent law.

FOR MORE INFORMATION OR TO REPORT A PROBLEM, you may contact the designated Privacy Officer, Assistant Athletic Trainer   If you feel your rights have been violated, you may file a complaint in writing with the designated Privacy Officer. If you are not satisfied with the resolution of the complaint, you may also file a complaint with the Secretary of Health and Human Services. You will not be retaliated against for filing a complaint.

(Continued...)

Konin JG, Frederick MA. *Documentation for Athletic Training*. Thorofare, NJ: SLACK Incorporated; 2005.

USE AND DISCLOSURE OF PROTECTED HEALTH INFORMATION

We may use or disclose your protected health information for treatment, payment and operations, and for purposes described below:

<u>We will use your health information for treatment</u>: e.g. we will use information obtained by a physician, nurse practitioner, nurse or other medical professionals, staff, trainees and volunteers in our office to determine your best course of treatment. The information obtained from you or from other providers will become part of your medical records. We may also disclose your health care information to other outside treating medical professionals and staff as deemed necessary for your care. For example, we may disclose your health information to an outside doctor for referral. We will also provide your health care providers with copies of various reports to assist him/her in your treatment. We will disclose personal health information to coaches pertaining to your current medical condition and any conditions that may restrict your ability to compete.

<u>We will use your health information for payment</u>: e.g. we may send a bill to you or to your insurance carrier. The information on or accompanying the bill may include information that identifies you, as well as your diagnosis, procedures, and supplies used as necessary to obtain payment.

<u>We will use your health information for regular health operations</u>: e.g. members of the medical staff, trainees, medical students, a Risk or Quality Improvement team, or similar internal operations may use your information to assess the care and outcomes of your care in an effort to improve the quality of the healthcare and service we provide or for educational purposes. For example, an internal review team may review your medical records to determine the appropriafeness of care. There may also be times in which our accountants, auditors or attorneys may be required to review your health information to meet their responsibilities.

<u>Other uses and disclosures not requiring authorization</u>

- <u>Business Associates</u>: There are some services provided in our organization through contracts with business associates, such as laboratory services and radiology services. We may disclose your health information to our business associate so that they can perform these services. To protect your health information, we require the business associate to appropriately safeguard your information.

- <u>Notification</u>: We may disclose your health information to a friend or family member involved in your care or assisting you in payment. We may also notify a family member, friend, or other person responsible for your care, about your location and general condition.

- <u>Disclosures required by law or for threats to safety</u>: We may disclose your health information as required by law, or if necessary to avert a serious threat to health or safety, although disclosures are limited if information is obtained through counseling or therapy.

- <u>Public Health</u>: As allowed by law, we may disclose your health information to public health or legal authorities to 1) prevent or control disease, injury or disability, 2) to report child abuse or domestic abuse, in which case you may be notified of the disclosure, 3) for purposes related to quality, safety, or effectiveness of FDA-regulated products or activity, 4) to identify exposure to, and prevent the spread of, communicable disease, including notification of individuals that may have been exposed to communicable disease, 5) to an employer to conduct medical surveillance of the workplace or to evaluate whether an employee has a work related illness or injury, 6) to health oversight agencies as provided by law and 7) to report births and deaths..

- <u>Law Enforcement and Court Proceedings</u>: We may disclose health information to law enforcement in the following circumstances 1) information required by law, 2) limited information for identification and location purposes, 3) information regarding suspected victims of crime, although we will usually attempt to first obtain your agreement to release the information, 4) information about a deceased individual if we have a suspicion that the death resulted from criminal conduct, 5) information that we believe in good faith establishes that a crime has been committed on our premises during our providing of emergency health care. We may also disclose health information to others as required by court or administrative order, or in response to a valid summons or subpoena, for civil subpoenas, we will seek assurances from the requesting party that reasonable efforts have been made to inform you of the subpoena.

- <u>Information Regarding Decedents</u>: We may disclose health information regarding a deceased person to: 1) coroners and medical examiners to identify cause of death or other duties, 2) funeral directors for their required duties and 3) to procurement organizations for purposes of organ and tissue donation.

(Continued...)

- Research: We may disclose health information to where you have authorized such disclosure. We may also disclose health information where the disclosure is solely for the purpose of designing a study, or where the disclosure concerns decedents, or the disclosure is approved by an institutional review board (IRB) or properly constituted Privacy Board if the Board has determined that obtaining authorization is not feasible and protocols are in place to ensure the privacy of your health information.

- Military, National Security and Correctional Department Disclosures: We may disclose health information in connection with the responsibilities of the armed services if you are a member, national security and intelligence, protective services for certain government officials, and to correctional officials for health and safety purposes if you are an inmate.

- Marketing and Appointment Reminders: We may contact you to provide appointment reminders or information about treatment alternative or other health related benefits and services that may be of interest to you.

- Fund raising: We may contact you as part of a fund raising effort.

Disclosures requiring authorization: All other disclosures of protected health information will only be made pursuant to your written authorization, which you have the right to revoke at any time, except to the extent we have already relied upon the authorization.

Federal law requires that we seek your acknowledgement of receipt of this Notice of Privacy Practices. Please sign below.

I acknowledge that I have received this Notice of Privacy Practices with and effective date of _____

Student-Athlete Signature:_____   **Date:** _____

If student-athlete is under 18:
Student-Athlete Representative Signature:_____   **Date:** _____

Description of Legal Guardianship: _____

Konin JG, Frederick MA. *Documentation for Athletic Training.* Thorofare, NJ: SLACK Incorporated; 2005.

Forest Institute Human Services Center

1322 S. Campbell * Springfield, MO 65807
Phone (417) 865-8943 * Fax (417) 831-6839
Authorization for Release of Information

Forest Institute Human Services Center
1322 S. Campbell
Springfield, MO 65807
(417) 865-8943

Name: _____ **DOB:** ___ / ___ / ___ **SSN:** ___ - ___ - ___

To:

_Southwest Missouri State University_____
_901 S. National, Springfield, MO 65804_____

I, the undersigned, do hereby authorize Forest Institute Human Services Center to _x_ release _x_ receive the following categories checked below regarding the above named individual.

X_ Assessment Information/Results   ___ Diagnosis
X_ Treatment Recommendations   X_ Treatment Progress
___ Results of Psychological Testing   ___ Progress Note(s)
___ Discharge Summary   X_ Drug Screen Results
___ Psychiatric Evaluation   ___ Medication History
X_ Other: _____
_____
_____

I understand that my records are protected under Federal Confidentiality Regulations and cannot be disclosed without my consent unless otherwise provided in the regulations. I also understand that I may revoke this consent except to the extent that action has been taken in reliance on it.

I hereby release any person, firm, physician, clinic, hospital or agency, public or private, from any liability for information furnished pursuant to this authorization. I waive my right to privileged communication and confidentiality to the Forest Institute Human Services Center.

The information to be released and/or received has been done by informed consent.

THE CONSENT EXPIRES ONE (1) YEAR FROM THE DATE OF AUTHORIZATION.

Authorized this _____ day of _____ in the year _____.

_____   _____
Signature of client or participant (or legal guardian or   Signature of witness
Authorized Representative if client is under 18 years
of age or has been adjudicated legally incompetent.)   _____
                                                             Signature of Clinic Director/Licensed Provider

Prohibition on redisclosure: This information has been disclosed to you from records for which confidentiality is protected by Federal Law. Federal regulations (42CFR Part 2) prohibit you from making any further disclosure of this information except with the specific written consent of the person to whom it pertains. A general authorization for the release of medical or other information, if held by another party, is not sufficient for this purpose. Federal regulations state that any person who violates any provision of this law shall be fined not more than $500 in the case of the first offense and not more than $5,000 in the case of each subsequent offense.

_____ Please mail the information described to:
Forest Institute Human services Center * 1322 S. Campbell * Springfield, MO 65807

Konin JG, Frederick MA. *Documentation for Athletic Training*. Thorofare, NJ: SLACK Incorporated; 2005.

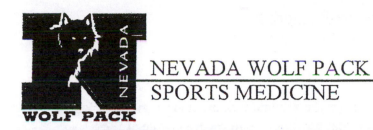

NEVADA WOLF PACK
SPORTS MEDICINE

Consent for Release of Medical Records

I _____, give my permission to release the stated portions of my medical records to _____.

_____

Please release the following information from my medical records:
_____ Entire Record
_____ Partial Record
Specify: _____

Recipient:
    Name _____
    Address _____
    _____
    _____
    Phone _____
    Email _____
    Fax _____

_____

I understand that this release will become effective on the day that it is signed and will continue to be in effect for 90 days. I also understand that I may cancel this release at any time by notifying the Nevada Sports Medicine staff in writing.

Signature _____ **Date** _____

Name _____ Phone _____
Address _____
_____

(Continued...)

Konin JG, Frederick MA. *Documentation for Athletic Training.* Thorofare, NJ: SLACK Incorporated; 2005.

Please read the following consent/authorization forms carefully:
(If you are under 18 years of age, your parents must also sign)

The basic consent of each is:

A.   Medical Consent: Allows the athletic trainers and team physician(s)
                                    to treat any injury you receive while at the
                                    University of Nevada.

B.   Authorization/Consent
      To Disclose Information: Allows those listed to release information to the
                                    NCAA, Conference, media and professional teams
                                    concerning your injuries/illness.

C.   Shared Responsibility   Acknowledges you that there are certain inherent
      for sport safety   risks involved in participating in intercollegiate
                                    athletics and that you are willing to assume
                                    responsibility for such risks.

D.   Aids & Intercollegiate   Acknowledges that HIV transmission is possible
      Athletics: through athletics.

If you should chose to refuse to sign any of these, please write **"Refuse to Sign"**, the
date, and your signature.

A photo copy of these authorizations shall be considered as effective and valid as the
original for the time I am a participant in the intercollegiate athletic program at the
University of Nevada.

FORMS
A.   Medical Consent

I hereby grant permission to the University of Nevada team physician(s) and/or the
consulting physician(s) to render to my son, daughter, or myself, any treatment or
medical or surgical care that they deem reasonably necessary to the health and well being
of the student athlete, including consults/referrals to outside medical professionals.

I also hereby authorize the athletic trainers at the University of Nevada who are under the
direction and guidance of the University of Nevada team physician(s) to render to my
son, daughter, or myself any preventative first aid, rehabilitation, or emergency treatment
that they deem reasonably necessary to the health and well being of the student athlete.

In case of serious injury or illness, I understand that reasonable effort will be made to
contact the parents/guardians. If contact cannot be made, I hereby give permission to the
University of Nevada sports medicine staff, other facilities, or health care providers to
administer emergency medical treatment including surgery as deemed advisable.

(Continued...)

Konin JG, Frederick MA. *Documentation for Athletic Training*. Thorofare, NJ: SLACK Incorporated; 2005.

I authorize the University of Nevada intercollegiate athletic department to provide the University of Nevada student health center any information requested, and authorize the University of Nevada student health center to provide the University of Nevada intercollegiate athletic department any information requested, concerning my health and athletic status.

Also, when necessary for executing such case, I grant permission for hospitalization at an accredited hospital.

I understand and agree that the University of Nevada may use or disclose protected health information for treatment, payment and operations in accordance with the Notice of Privacy Practices that I have received, and any posted amendments to that Notice. I understand that the University of Nevada will not use or disclose protected health information for any purpose other than treatment, payment and healthcare operations, unless such person or entity is authorized to receive such information under law or I have provided a written authorization. (*See full explanation of disclosures and rights in the Notice of Privacy Practices*) If I am being treated while I am a student athlete, I consent and agree that my health information may be used and disclosed in accordance with the Notice of Privacy Practices (and any posted revision of that Notice) and the federal Health Insurance Portability and Accountability Act (HIPAA).

Date:_____   _____
                                        Signature

Signature may be that of athlete 18 years
of age and over: if under 18, please   _____
have parent or guardian sign.   Social Security Number

                                              _____
                                              Parent or Guardian

B. Consent/Authorization for Disclosure of Information

I, _____, hereby authorize the University of Nevada
        Name of Student Athlete
and its coaches, physicians, athletic trainers and health care personnel to disclose my protected health information and any related information regarding any injury or illness during my training for, and participation in, intercollegiate athletics to the NCAA, my institution's athletic conference, to media outlets (including the University of Nevada Sports Information Office), to professional sports teams, and to their respective employees or agents.

I understand that my protected health information will be used by the NCAA, Conference, media, and/or professional sports teams for the purpose of statistical reporting, providing to the public information regarding the general type of any injury or illness that I have incurred, the medical professionals involved in my care, the current status of my health, and my probable return date to active participation, and providing

(Continued...)

Konin JG, Frederick MA. *Documentation for Athletic Training*. Thorofare, NJ: SLACK Incorporated; 2005.

professional sports teams with medical/health information and records for player evaluation purposes.

I understand that my injury/illness information is protected by federal regulations under either the Health Information Portability and Accountability Act (HIPAA) or the Family Educational Rights and Privacy Act of 1974 (the Buckley Amendment) and may not be disclosed without either my authorization under HIPAA or my consent under the Buckley Amendment. I understand that my signing of this authorization/consent is voluntary and that my institution will not condition any health care treatment or payment, enrollment in a health plan or receipt of any benefits (if applicable) on whether I provide the consent/authorization requested. I also understand that I am not required to sign this authorization/consent in order to be eligible to participate in NCAA or conference athletics.

I also understand that the NCAA, Conference, media, and professional teams may not be covered by the Buckley Amendment or HIPAA and that these regulations may not apply to their use or disclosure of my injury/illness information.

This authorization/consent expires 380 days from the date of my signature below, but I have the right to revoke it in writing at any time by sending written notification to the athletic director at my institution. I understand that a revocation is not effective to the extent action has already been taken in reliance on this authorization/consent.

_____   _____
            Signature   Date

If under age 18:

_____   _____
Signature of Parent or Guardian (identify which)   Date

C.   Shared Responsibility for Sport Safety

Participation in sport requires an acceptance of risk of injury. Athletes rightfully assume that those who are responsible for the conduce of sport have taken reasonable precaution to minimize such risk and that their peers participating in the sport will not intentionally inflict injury upon them.

Periodic analysis of injury patterns and refinements in the rules and other safety decisions in an ongoing process. However to legislate safety via a rule book and equipment standards, while often necessary, seldom is effective by itself; and to rely on officials to enforce compliance with the rule book is an insufficient as to rely on warning labels to produce compliance with safety guidelines. "Compliance" means respect on everyone's part for the intent and purpose of a rule or guideline.

I understand that by voluntarily participating in athletics at collegiate level, I am undertaking a non-controllable risk which may result in an injury that may be very severe in nature. Such an injury may result in paralysis and/or death. It is further my understanding that it is entirely my responsibility to report any illness or injury to the

(Continued...)

Konin JG, Frederick MA. *Documentation for Athletic Training.* Thorofare, NJ: SLACK Incorporated; 2005.

athletic training staff or team physician(s). If I do not the University of Nevada will not be responsible for those injuries. A student participating in intercollegiate athletics who reports to a physician without the knowledge of the certified athletic trainer in charge will accept the personal responsibility and expenses of such action. Exceptions are made for away games and during the absence of the athletic trainer at the time of the accident/emergency. I also understand that I must refrain from practice or play while ill or injured. The full-time athletic training staff, through the direction of the team physician(s) will inform the athlete and respective coaching staff of all athlete's injuries and playing/practicing status.

All walk-on student-athletes MUST have primary insurance coverage that is applicable in the state of Nevada. The University of Nevada athletic insurance policy provides insurance coverage for injuries sustained while participating in play or practice and is "EXCESS COVERAGE ONLY". This means that it pays benefits only after taking into consideration the insurance plan held by you or your parent(s). Illness and injuries not directly associated with athletic participation are the responsibility of the student athlete.

I understand sickness and/or injuries are common in all athletics and that the University of Nevada Intercollegiate Athletic Department will provide the most reasonable medical coverage in order to reduce the severity of such illness and/or injuries. The administration, coaches, athletic trainer, and managers will equally provide to each student, equipment required to produce the safest possible intercollegiate athletic environment regardless of age, sex, race, or religion.

I understand that the athletic medical insurance does not cover me until I have been cleared by an athletic medical physical examination. I further understand that the University of Nevada athletic medical insurance is for coverage of athletic injuries/illnesses that are directly related to participation in intercollegiate athletics.

I have read the following (pertains to football only)

> **WARNING:** Do not use this helmet to butt, ram or spear opposing players. This is a violation of the football rules and can result in severe head, brain or neck injury, paralysis, or death to you and possible injury to your opponent. There is a risk to you and possible injury to your opponent. There is a risk that injuries may occur as a result of accidental contact without intent to butt, ram or spear. NO HELMET CAN PREVENT ALL SUCH INJURIES. (This information can be found inside every helmet and should be read daily.)

I have been instructed on and issued all necessary equipment that is standard of the NCAA rules.
I have read the above shared responsibility statement and understand that there are certain inherent risks involved in participating in intercollegiate athletics. I acknowledge the fact

(Continued...)

Konin JG, Frederick MA. *Documentation for Athletic Training*. Thorofare, NJ: SLACK Incorporated; 2005.

that these risks exist and I am willing to assume responsibility for such risks while participating at the University of Nevada.

Date:_____

_____
Signature

Signature may be that of athlete over 18 years of age: if under 18, please have parent or guardian sign.

_____
Social Security Number

_____
Parent or Guardian

D.   AIDS AND INTERCOLLEGIATE ATHLETICS

The Acquired Immunodeficiency Syndrome (AIDS) is caused by a virus or HIV (Human Immunodeficiency Virus). HIV has been isolated in blood, semen, vaginal secretions, saliva, tears, breast milk, cerebrospinal fluid, amniotic fluid, and urine. However, available evidence has implicated only blood, semen, vaginal secretion, and possibly breast milk in the transmission of HIV.

The risk of infection is increased by having multiple sex partners, unprotected sex, and in sharing needles among intravenous drug users.

Although the precise risks of transmission during exposure of open wounds or mucous membrane contaminated blood is not known, theoretically there is a possibility of HIV transmission by blood from one student-athlete to an open wound of another student-athlete.

Therefore, the intercollegiate athletic department, team precautions as recommended by the Center of Disease Control in care of all student-athletes, since medical history and examination cannot reliably verify HIV infected patients.

In addition the Student Health Center on campus will provide HIV testing (fee required) to all students who so request. Information on testing dates may be obtained in the University of Nevada Sports Medicine Center for athletes or by calling the Student Health Center at 784-6598.

Date:_____

_____
Signature

Signature may be that of athlete over 18 years of age: if under 18, please have parent or guardian sign.

_____
Social Security Number

_____
Parent or Guardian

Konin JG, Frederick MA. *Documentation for Athletic Training*. Thorofare, NJ: SLACK Incorporated; 2005.

Medical Release Form

Student Athlete's Name (Print)_____ Sport _____ Date_____

Date of Birth _____ Social Security # _____

Campus Phone_____ Campus Address_____
                                                    Street   City, State, Zip

Permission to Treat Statement

Permission is hereby granted to Salisbury University to proceed with any needed medical treatment deemed necessary in the event the parent or guardian cannot be contacted. In the event of serious illness, the need for major surgery or significant accident or injury, I understand an attempt will be made to contact me in an expeditious manner. In the event I cannot be contacted, permission is granted to render all treatment necessary in the best interest of the above-named athlete.

_____   _____   _____
Parent/Guardian Name (Print)   Parent/Guardian Signature   Date

_____   _____   _____
Relationship to Student Athlete   Home Phone   Work Phone

_____
Parent/Guardian Address   Street   City, State, Zip

Permission to Obtain Medical Records

I hereby give the Salisbury University medical staff permission to obtain medical records pertaining to any injury or condition incurred while participating in intercollegiate athletics at Salisbury University. I understand an attempt will be made to inform me of the necessity of obtaining medical records.

_____   Date   _____
Athlete's Signature

Permission for Medical Records Release to Parent/Guardian

I hereby give the Salisbury University medical staff permission to release my medical record/information to my parent/guardian. I understand an attempt will be made to inform me of any release of medical record/information.

Athlete's Signature _____   Date   _____

Permission for Medical Records Release to Coaching Staff and Athletic Officials

I hereby give the Salisbury University medical staff permission to release pertinent medical information to the Salisbury University intercollegiate coaching staff and athletic officials. I understand an attempt will be made to inform me of any release of medical record/information.

Athlete's Signature _____   Date   _____

AGREEMENT TO PARTICIPATE FOR ATHLETES WITH THE LOSS OF A PAIRED ORGAN

I,_____(name), wish to participate in intercollegiate athletics, and more particularly, the _____(name of sport) program at Southwest Missouri State University. In connection with my participation, I acknowledge the risk of possible physical harm to me as a result of my participation is increased because of my loss of a paired organ_____(missing organ) which I sustained in the past, and for which I have received medical attention. While there is no immediate danger to me, I am told that strenuous, collision type activities, such as _____(name of sport) could render me more susceptible to future problems with my remaining_____(missing organ) than might normally be expected.

I have discussed alternative activities to participation in_____ (name of sport) with the head coach, athletic trainer and the physician who conducted the pre-participation physical examination. I have discussed the situation with my parents and we understand the potential danger of participation in_____(name of sport).

Notwithstanding that my participation in intercollegiate_____ (name of sport) constitutes more risk to me than it does other athletes, I nevertheless wish to participate in intercollegiate_____(name of sport) at Southwest Missouri State University. In making this decision, I am aware of the value of intercollegiate athletics in my life, and choose to continue my participation in order to take advantage of those values. In weighing the risk to myself of potential injury now and in the future, I wish to exonerate and save harmless Southwest Missouri State University, its agents and employees, the athletic staff of Southwest Missouri State University, the physicians and other practitioners of the healing arts treating me, from any and all liability as a result of injury to my _____(missing organ) which hereinafter may be claimed as a result of my participation of the program of the college, or any treatment by any of the foregoing physicians of any conditions or injuries sustained by me in the past to my _____ _____(missing organ)and to any injury that may occur in the future which is unrelated to my previous injury. I execute this agreement freely, fully intending to be bound by the same.

_____
STUDENT-ATHLETE

Signature may be that of athlete over 18 years of age; if under 18, please have it signed by parent or guardian.

_____
SOCIAL SECURITY NUMBER

_____
PARENT OR GUARDIAN

Date:_____

Konin JG, Frederick MA. *Documentation for Athletic Training.* Thorofare, NJ: SLACK Incorporated; 2005.

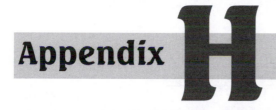

Appendix H

COMMONLY USED FORMS—
EVALUATION FORMS

These forms are predesigned and used to document findings from evaluations performed at given times, to specific joints or pertaining to a general medical condition.

CONTENTS

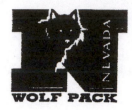

University of Nevada
Athletic Training
Injury Follow-up and Progress Notes

Name:_____   Sport:_____

Injury: _____   DOI:_____

_____
_____

Date:___/___/___

_____
_____
_____
_____
_____

Date:___/___/___

_____
_____
_____
_____
_____

Date:___/___/___

_____
_____
_____
_____
_____

Date:___/___/___

_____
_____
_____
_____
_____

Date:___/___/___

_____
_____
_____
_____
_____

UNIVERSITY OF NEVADA
SPORTS MEDICINE
CASHELL FIELDHOUSE/265
RENO, NEVADA 89557-0094

PHONE: 775-784-4045
FAX: 775-784-8077

Konin JG, Frederick MA. *Documentation for Athletic Training*. Thorofare, NJ: SLACK Incorporated; 2005.

Jones Athletic Training Department
Athlete Rehabilitation Form

Name:_____   **Date:**_____

Sport:_____   **Injury:**_____

Goal Setting

Short Term Goals:

1. _____   2. _____

3. _____   4. _____

Long Term Goals:

1. _____   2. _____

3. _____   4. _____

Rehabilitation Progress Notes

Date	Athletic Trainer	Comments	Home Instructions

Konin JG, Frederick MA. *Documentation for Athletic Training*. Thorofare, NJ: SLACK Incorporated; 2005.

INJURY EVALUATION – SHOULDER

WOLF PACK

Name:_____   Sport:_____   DOI:_____   Site:_____

Game – Practice – Wt. Room – Conditioning – Other   Cont. play – DNF   Surface:_____

Body Part: L R BiL _____   Type of Injury: Acute Chronic Re-Injury

HISTORY / MECHANISM OF INJURY:

Direct Blow: Location_____   Instability: Ant. / Post. / Inferior

Forced Flexion / Extension   Forced Ext. / Int. Rotation   Forced Abduction / Adduction

Other:_____

OBSERVATION:

General Appearance:_____

Edema: WNL Mild / Mod / Severe   Location: _____

Eccymosis: WNL Mild / Mod / Severe Location: _____

Deformity: WNL Mild / Mod / Severe Location: _____

PALPATION:

Bony Structures: WNL or Pain w/palpation Location: _____

Soft Tissue: WNL or Pain w/palpation   Location: _____

RANGE OF MOTION:

AROM: Shoulder Flexion: WNL or Decreased   Shoulder Extension: WNL or Decreased
Shoulder Abduction: WNL or Decreased   Shoulder Adduction: WNL or Decreased
Shoulder Internal Rot: WNL or Decreased   Shoulder External Rot: WNL or Decreased
Shoulder Elevation: WNL or Decreased   Shoulder Depression: WNL or Decreased
Shoulder Protraction: WNL or Decreased   Shoulder Retraction: WNL or Decreased

PROM   Shoulder Flexion: WNL or Decreased   Shoulder Extension: WNL or Decreased
Shoulder Abduction: WNL or Decreased   Shoulder Adduction: WNL or Decreased
Shoulder Internal Rot: WNL or Decreased   Shoulder External Rot: WNL or Decreased
Shoulder Elevation: WNL or Decreased   Shoulder Depression: WNL or Decreased
Shoulder Protraction: WNL or Decreased   Shoulder Retraction: WNL or Decreased

RROM: Shoulder Flexion: WNL or Decreased-Grade_____   Shoulder Extension: WNL or Decreased-Grade_____
Shoulder Abduction: WNL or Decreased-Grade_____   Shoulder Adduction: WNL or Decreased-Grade_____
Shoulder Internal Rot: WNL or Decreased-Grade_____ Shoulder External Rot: WNL or Decreased-Grade_____
Shoulder Elevation: WNL or Decreased-Grade_____   Shoulder Depression: WNL or Decreased-Grade_____
Shoulder Protraction: WNL or Decreased-Grade_____ Shoulder Retraction: WNL or Decreased-Grade_____

OTHER:_____

SPECIAL TESTS:

Apprehension: Pos / Neg in IR / ER   Ant / Post Instability: Pos / Neg   Impingement: Pos / Neg

Empty Can: Pos / Neg   Speeds: Pos / Neg   Biceps Tendon: Pos / Neg   Adson's: Pos / Neg

Other:_____

ASSESSMENT:_____

SIGNATURE: Certified Athletic Trainer: _____   Date:_____
Student Athletic Trainer: _____   Date:_____

(Continued...)

Konin JG, Frederick MA. *Documentation for Athletic Training.* Thorofare, NJ: SLACK Incorporated; 2005.

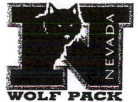

WOLF PACK

INJURY EVALUATION – SHOULDER

PLAN: Ice   Stabilize   Transport via: EMS / Personal Auto / AT Escort to_____
        Modalities: E-Stim   Ultrasound   Cryotherapy / Cryostretch
        Exercises: PNF   MRE,s   PRE's
        Other:_____

_____

_____

REFERRAL: ROC – Physician _____   Date of Referral: _____
           NPT – Therapist _____   Date of Referral: _____
           Other - _____

NOTES / FOLLOW UP:
    Date:_____

_____

_____

_____

_____

    Date:_____

_____

_____

_____

    Date:_____

_____

_____

_____

    Date:_____

_____

_____

_____

    Date:_____

_____

_____

_____

    Date:_____

_____

_____

_____

    Date:_____

_____

_____

_____

Konin JG, Frederick MA. *Documentation for Athletic Training*. Thorofare, NJ: SLACK Incorporated; 2005.

Knee Evaluation

Name:_____ Sport:_____ Date:_____

BP:_____ HR:_____ Practice____ Game____ Evaluator:_____

HISTORY

a. Do you remember a specific episode of trauma? If yes, when and please describe._____

_____

    If no, do you remember when you began to feel the discomfort? How long?_____

    Has it progressively gotten worse?_____

    b. Have you ever had any other injuries to this body part, knee or patella. If yes, then when and how many

    times?_____

    Did you recover? Is it worse than before?_____

c. Did you hear or feel a pop/ have a sense of giving away?_____

d. Do you feel any crepitus/grinding/popping?_____

    Does your knee lock up on occasions?_____

e. Do you ever have swelling or puffing around the knee joint?_____

f. Can you put your finger on the point that gives you the most pain?_____

g. At the time of your injury, describe the pain?_____

    Dull, diffuse, burning throbbing, aching, sharp, knife-like?_____

h. Do you have pain or discomfort walking up stairs?_____

    Do you have pain or discomfort walking down stairs_____

    Do you have pain slowing down from a run or fast walk?_____

i. Has the pain changed? Yes or no?____ How?_____ Timespan_____

    Rate it on a scale of 0 to 10 (with 0 being none and 10 being excrutiating)_____

j. What have you done since the injury?_____

k. What makes the pain worse/what makes it better?_____

l. Does pain wake you up at night?_____

m. Do you have stiffness in your knee in the morning, after awakening?_____

n. Do you have pain in any other parts of the body? Is it referred?_____

o. Were you taped or wrapped?_____

p. What type of shoe were you wearing?_____ Did your shoes have a cleat?_____

q. Do you wear any type of foot support? _____ How long have you worn them?_____

r. Have you made a change in terrain/training regimen?_____

OBSERVATION

a. Condition of athlete? (Excellent - Good - Fair - Poor)_____

b. Observe weight-description:_____

c. Observe gait? (Non-weight bearing - Partial weight bearing - Full weight bearing)_____

d. Observe Limp? (Pronounced - Mild - Slight - Unable to bear weight)_____

e. Gross deformity-description:_____

f. Swelling?   (Hemarthrosis - moderate - mild effusion)_____

g. Discoloration? (echymosis and location)_____

h. Supinated/pronated feet? (Positive - Negative) description_____

i. Heel cord tightness? (Positive - Negative) description_____

j. Hamstring tightness? (Positive - Negative) description_____

k. Patella Alignment? patella alta_____ patella baja_____ patella lateral_____

l. Quadriceps: VMO dysplasia_____

m. Girth Measurements? Involved: _____ 3" _____ 6" _____ 9" Non Involved _____ 3" _____ 6" _____ 9"

n. Tibial Torsion? yes/no   (Bi lateral___ Unilateral____)

o. Varas knee? yes/no   Valgus knee? yes/no

p. Recurvatum? yes/no   (Bi Lateral____ Unilateral____)

q. Angle of Patella: _____ right _____ left

PALPATION RULE OUT A FRACTURE

(POSITIVE - NEGATIVE) COMPRESSION_____ PERCUSSION_____ DISTRACTION_____

	Tender	Crepits		Tender	Crepitus		Tender	Crepitus
1. vastus medialis	yes/no	yes/no	2. rectus femoris	yes/no	yes/no	3. patella	yes/no	yes/no
4. superior medial pol	yes/no	yes/no	5. superior lateral pole	yes/no	yes/no	6 .inferior pole	yes/no	yes/no
7. tibial tuberosity	yes/no	yes/no	8 .infrapatellar tendon	yes/no	yes/no	9. medial tibial plateau	yes/no	yes/no
10. medial meniscus	yes/no	yes/no	11. .medial femoral con.	yes/no	yes/no	12. medial collateral ligament	yes/no	yes/no
13. adductor musculature	yes/no	yes/no	14. lateral tibial plateau	yes/no	yes/no	15. lateral meniscus yes/no	yes/no	
16. lateral meniscus	yes/no	yes/no	17. lateral joint line	yes/no	yes/no	18. head of the fibula	yes/no	yes/no
19. lateral collateral lig.	yes/no	yes/no	20. abductor musculatrue	yes/no	yes/no	21. biceps femoris	yes/no	yes/no
22.semitendinosus	yes/no	yes/no	23.semimembranosus	yes/no	yes/no	24.popliteal fossa	yes/no	yes/no
25.gastrocnemius	yes/no	yes/no						

(Continued...)

Konin JG, Frederick MA. *Documentation for Athletic Training.* Thorofare, NJ: SLACK Incorporated; 2005.

ASSESSING MOTION

	General ROM	Goniometer	End Feel	Muscle Testing w/Gravity	Muscle testing w/out Gravity
Flexion (0-135)	_____	_____	_____	_____	_____
Extension	_____	_____	_____	_____	_____

RATINGS

General ROM	(Painfull-Limited-Full)
Goniometer	(Prcentage of Angle)
End Feel	Normal (Bony - Soft Tissue Apposition - Soft Tissue Stretch - Capsular Stretch)
	Abnormal (Hard - Soft- - Firm - Springy Block - Empty - Spasm)
Muscle Testing w/Gravity	(5 4 4- 3+ 3 3- 2+)
Muscle Testing w/out Gravity	(2 2- 1+ 1 0)

STRESS TESTS

(+1   +2   +3)

Patella Tend/Lig. Length Test	L__ R__	Patellar Aprrehension Test	L__ R__	Patella Tap Test	L__ R__
Q Angle Test	L__ R__	Medial/Lateral Grind Test	L__ R__	Bounce Home Test	L__ R__
Patellar Grind Test	L__ R__	Renne Test	L__ R__	Noble Test L__ R__
Hughston's Plica Test	L__ R__	Godfrey 90/90	L__ R__	Posterior Sag Test L__ R__
Reverse Pivot Shift Test	L__ R__	Anterior Lachman Test	L__ R__	Anterior Drawer Test L__ R__
Slocum Test IR	L__ R__	Slocum Test ER	L__ R__	Pivot Shift Test L__ R__
Posterior Drawer Test	L__ R__	Posteromedial Drawer Test	L__ R__	Posteriorlateral Drawer L__ R__
Posterior Lachman Test	L__ R__	External Rotation Recurvatum	L__ R__	Valgus Stress Test L__ R__
Varus Stress Test	L__ R__	Jerk Test	L__ R__	McMurray Test L__ R__
Apley Compression Test	L__ R__				

NEUROLOGICAL EXAM
(POSITIVE - NEGATIVE)

NERVE ROOT LEVEL	SENSORY TESTING	MOTOR TESTING	REFLEX TESTING
L2	_____	_____	_____
L3	_____	_____	_____
L4	_____	_____	_____
L5	_____	_____	
S1	_____	_____	

CIRCULATORY EXAM
(POSITIVE - NEGATIVE)

Popliteal Pulse_____

FUNCTIONAL TESTS

Weight bearing_____
Stand on injured extremity_____
Walk_____
Hop on both feet_____
Hop on injured extremity_____
Straight line jog_____
Full speed run to a dead stop_____
Carioca to left/right_____
Large figure-8 and make progressively smaller and faster_____
Full sprint with 90 degree cuts_____
Sports specific movements_____
All movements pain free/ no limp_____

NOTES

Impression:_____
_____
Referral: Emergency Room_____

Physician's Office_____
Acute Management: Crutches___   Posterior Splint___   Compression Bandage___   Air Caist ___   Vacuum Splint___   Speedi Splint___
X-rays: Anterior/Posterior view_____
         Lateral view_____
         Mortis view _____
         Anterior/Posterior view with stress_____

Konin JG, Frederick MA. *Documentation for Athletic Training*. Thorofare, NJ: SLACK Incorporated; 2005.

NEVADA FOOTBALL
INJURY REPORTING SHEET

Date:_____   Uniform:_____   Surface:_____

( ) Dict._____   ( ) Dict._____   ( ) Dict._____
Name:_____   Name:_____   Name:_____
Injury:_____   Injury:_____   Injury:_____
Type:_____   Type:_____   Type:_____
Drill: Drill: Drill:
Contact / Non   Contact / Non   Contact / Non
Injury: Injury: Injury:
Contact / Non   Contact / Non   Contact / Non
Cont / DNF   Cont / DNF   Cont / DNF

( ) Dict._____   ( ) Dict._____   ( ) Dict._____
Name:_____   Name:_____   Name:_____
Injury:_____   Injury:_____   Injury:_____
Type:_____   Type:_____   Type:_____
Drill: Drill: Drill:
Contact / Non   Contact / Non   Contact / Non
Injury: Injury: Injury:
Contact / Non   Contact / Non   Contact / Non
Cont / DNF   Cont / DNF   Cont / DNF

( ) Dict._____   ( ) Dict._____   ( ) Dict._____
Name:_____   Name:_____   Name:_____
Injury:_____   Injury:_____   Injury:_____
Type:_____   Type:_____   Type:_____
Drill: Drill: Drill:
Contact / Non   Contact / Non   Contact / Non
Injury: Injury: Injury:
Contact / Non   Contact / Non   Contact / Non
Cont / DNF   Cont / DNF   Cont / DNF

( ) Dict._____   ( ) Dict._____   ( ) Dict._____
Name:_____   Name:_____   Name:_____
Injury:_____   Injury:_____   Injury:_____
Type:_____   Type:_____   Type:_____
Drill: Drill: Drill:
Contact / Non   Contact / Non   Contact / Non
Injury: Injury: Injury:
Contact / Non   Contact / Non   Contact / Non
Cont / DNF   Cont / DNF   Cont / DNF

Konin JG, Frederick MA. *Documentation for Athletic Training.* Thorofare, NJ: SLACK Incorporated; 2005.

Home Rehabilitation Program

_____

Name: _____ Sport: _____

Injury/Illness: _____

Home Phone: _____ Email: _____

Supervising Certified Athletic Trainer: _____

ATC Phone: _____ ATC Email: _____

The exercises listed below should be performed _____ time(s) a day. The supervising certified athletic trainer will communicate frequently with you while you are away from school. However, if at any times you have questions or concerns, you should contact the supervising certified athletic trainer as soon as possible. It is your responsibility to perform these exercises as prescribed so that you have an optimal rehabilitation outcome following your injury/illness.

Exercises to be performed:

1. _____

2. _____

3. _____

4. _____

5. _____

☐ Additional information provided on attached document

Konin JG, Frederick MA. *Documentation for Athletic Training*. Thorofare, NJ: SLACK Incorporated; 2005.

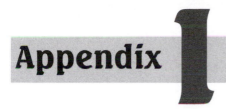

Appendix 1

COMMONLY USED FORMS— MISCELLANEOUS FORMS

Many forms can be designed to facilitate thorough, efficient, and necessary documentation. A few examples are provided here that pertain to fax cover sheets, research consent forms, weight classification documents, emergency action plans, medical referrals, and professional goal setting.

CONTENTS

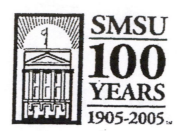

www.smsu.edu/centennial

Fax Cover Sheet

Date:

Athletic Training Services
Southwest Missouri State University
901 South National Avenue, Springfield, MO 65804

To: _____   **From:** _____

Fax: _____   **Pages:** (including cover sheet) _____

Phone: _____   **Date:** _____

Re: _____   **CC:** _____

☐ **Urgent**   ☐ **For Review**   ☐ **Please Comment**   ☐ **Please Reply**   ☐ **Please Recycle**

• **NOTICE OF CONFIDENTIALITY:** The documents accompanying this facsimile transmission contain confidential information belonging to the sender which is legally and/or medically privileged. The information is intended only for the use of the individual or entity named above. If you are not the intended recipient, you are hereby notified that any disclosure, copying, distribution or taking of any action on the contents of this facsimile information is strictly prohibited. **If you have received this facsimile transmission in error, please immediately notify us by telephone to arrange for return of the documents to us.**

COMMENTS:

James Madison University
Sports Medicine
Godwin Hall, MSC 2301
Harrisonburg, VA 22807

Phone: 540-568
Fax: 540-568-

Attention: _____   Fax: _____

To: _____   Date: _____

From: _____   Total Pages: _____
                                 (Including this page)
Subject: _____

_____

Message:

The document(s) accompanying this transmission contain information from the Department of
Sports Medicine at James Madison University. This information is intended only for the use of the
individual or entity named as the written recipient on this cover sheet. All information provided
within this fax transmission is considered private and confidential. Therefore, if you are in receipt of
this transmission and are not the written named recipient you are hereby notified that any
disclosure, copying and/or distribution of this information is strictly prohibited. If you have received
this fax in error, please notify our office immediately by telephone at (540) 568-6562. Thank you for
your assistance.

Konin JG, Frederick MA. *Documentation for Athletic Training.* Thorofare, NJ: SLACK Incorporated; 2005.

INITIAL MINIMUM WRESTLING WEIGHT CLASSIFICATION

Must be completed by medical personnel performing student's physical evaluation.

Initial Minimum Wrestling Weight Classification for _____
                                                                                    (Name)

Enrolled in _____ School

I certify that the herein named student may wrestle at the following **initial** minimum weight classification:

(medical examiner circle and initial one)

SENIOR HIGH SCHOOL (Fourteen Weight Classifications):

| 103 lbs. | 112 lbs. | 119 lbs. | 125 lbs. | 130 lbs. | 135 lbs. | 140 lbs. |
| 145 lbs. | 152 lbs. | 160 lbs. | 171 lbs. | 189 lbs. | 215 lbs. | 275 lbs. |

JUNIOR HIGH/MIDDLE SCHOOL (Eighteen Weight Classifications):

| 75 lbs. | 80 lbs. | 85 lbs. | 90 lbs. | 95 lbs. | 100 lbs. | 105 lbs. | 110 lbs. | 115 lbs. |
| 122 lbs. | 130 lbs. | 138 lbs. | 145 lbs. | 155 lbs. | 165 lbs. | 185 lbs. | 210 lbs. | 250 lbs. |

Name of Medical Examiner:_____Date:_____

Address:_____Phone:_____

Signature MD, DO, PAC, CRNP, SNP _____

Recommended Tests:

Water weighing

Caliper measurement

Other accepted tests

Konin JG, Frederick MA. *Documentation for Athletic Training*. Thorofare, NJ: SLACK Incorporated; 2005.

Research Involving Student Athletes

Individuals conducting research at James Madison University must have their proposals approved by the Institution Review Board (IRB). At times, proposals may be approved that involve subjects who also happen to be student athletes. It is possible that while the nature of a proposal that includes student athletes as subjects may be approved in scope by the IRB, the timing of performing the data collection may not be entirely conducive to the student athlete and he or she's athletic participation schedule. As such, a recommendation is being made to allow for the Director of Sports Medicine and various individuals within the athletic department to review each proposal prior to granting full approval.

The following protocol is suggested;

1. Proposals for research involving student athletes should be forwarded to the Director of Sports Medicine. The Director of Sports Medicine will review the proposal with the Team Physician, appropriate head coach of the sport involved, and others necessary (i.e., strength coach, athletic student advising) depending upon the scope of the proposal.
2. Proposals should include specific information regarding the scope of the study, purpose, benefits, risks, nature of activity, dates to be performed, length of time needed per subject, safety issues, individuals responsible for performing the study, and all other information required by the IRB for general proposal purposes. **Proposals should only be forwarded once approved by the IRB**.
3. The proposal will either be approved as is, approved with suggested modifications, or rejected with rationale. Once reviewed, the researcher(s) will receive written notification. No study may begin using student athletes as subjects until written approval is granted.

The Athletics Department would like to encourage collaboration with academic endeavors and encourages researchers to promote study in the area of intercollegiate athletics. By working together, we will ensure that each student athlete is able to achieve maximal benefits from participation in intercollegiate athletics at James Madison University.

Konin JG, Frederick MA. *Documentation for Athletic Training*. Thorofare, NJ: SLACK Incorporated; 2005.

Protocol Checklist for Research Involving Student Athletes

Name of Researcher(s) _____   Date _____

_____

Phone: _____ Fax: _____ Email: _____

Mailing Address: _____

_____

Title of Research: _____

_____

Date(s) research to be conducted: _____

Items forwarded to Director of Sports Medicine:

☐   Original Proposal
☐   Copy of IRB Approval Letter
☐   Copy of Subject's Consent To Participate Form

Following review of the submitted proposal for research involving student athletes, the work has been:

☐   Accepted as proposed

☐   Accepted with modifications: _____

    _____

☐   Denied on the basis of: _____

    _____

_____   _____
Director of Sports Medicine   Date

_____   _____
Director of Compliance   Date

_____   _____
Head Coach   Date

_____   _____
                                                     Date

Konin JG, Frederick MA. *Documentation for Athletic Training*. Thorofare, NJ: SLACK Incorporated; 2005.

FOOTBALL PRACTICE FIELD
EMERGENCY ACTION PLAN

Location: FB practice field / Intramural fields @ the University of Nevada

Phone Locations: Training Room inside Cashell Field House
Nevada Physical Therapy inside Sports Medicine Complex

1. State Name and where are calling from:
        My name is _____. I am an athletic trainer at the University of
Nevada. I am calling from _____ at the University of Nevada.

2. State the nature of injury or condition:
        We have a possible _____. State level of consciousness and if
athlete has a stable BP and pulse.

3. State the location of the athlete (be as specific as possible):
        The athlete is _____.

4. Give the following directions:
        A. Go north on Virginia St. Turn right onto campus south of Lawlor Events
Center. At the stop sign turn left, and go straight up the hill past Cashell Field House on
your left. At the next stop sign turn left, then immediately right at the tennis courts east
of the football stadium. Proceed to the grass practice fields east of the tennis courts.
There will be someone there to direct the paramedics.
        B. Go south on Virginia St. from North McCarran. Turn left onto campus south of
Lawlor Events Center. At the stop sign turn left, and go straight up the hill past Cashell
Field House on your left. At the next stop sign turn left, then immediately right at the
tennis courts east of the football stadium. Proceed to the grass practice fields east of the
tennis courts. There will be someone there to direct the paramedics.

* Location of athlete will determine which set of directions to give.

5. Do not hang up until you are told to do so.

Konin JG, Frederick MA. *Documentation for Athletic Training*. Thorofare, NJ: SLACK Incorporated; 2005.

MACKAY STADIUM / TRACK
EMERGENCY ACTION PLAN

Location: Mackay Stadium @ the University of Nevada

Phone Locations: Pay phone by bathrooms at southwest corner of stadium
Training Room & Weight Room inside Cashell Field House

1. State Name and where are calling from:
My name is _____. I am an athletic trainer at the University of Nevada. I am calling from Mackay Stadium / Cashell Field House at the University of Nevada.

2. State the nature of injury or condition:
We have a possible _____. State level of consciousness and if athlete has a stable BP and pulse.

3. State the location of the athlete (be as specific as possible):
The athlete is <u>(on the football field, track, etc.)</u>

4. Give the following directions:
A. Go north on Virginia St. Turn right onto campus south of Lawlor Events Center. At the stop sign turn left and go up the hill. Turn left towards main entrance to stadium and go past the brick building. Turn right into gate #2 at the southwest corner of the stadium. There will be someone there to direct the paramedics.
B. Go north on Virginia St. Turn right onto campus south of Lawlor Events Center. At the stop sign turn left, and go straight up the hill past Cashell Field House on your left. At the next stop sign turn left and into gate #10 at the southeast corner of the stadium. There will be someone there to direct the paramedics.
C. Go south on Virginia St. from North McCarran. Turn left onto campus south of Lawlor Events Center. At the stop sign turn left and go up the hill. Turn left towards main entrance to stadium and go past the brick building. Turn right into gate #2 at the southwest corner of the stadium. There will be someone there to direct the paramedics.

* Location of athlete will determine which set of directions to give.

5. Do not hang up until you are told to do so.

Konin JG, Frederick MA. *Documentation for Athletic Training*. Thorofare, NJ: SLACK Incorporated; 2005.

ATHLETIC TRAINING SERVICES
Southwest Missouri State University

PRE-OPERATIVE INSTRUCTION FOR OUTPATIENT SURGERY

INSTRUCTIONS TO PATIENT:

1. <u>NO MILK OR SOLIDS</u> for 8 hours and <u>NO CLEAR LIQUIDS</u> for 3 hours prior to surgery. (Clear liquids = water, apple juice, tea and coffee without milk.

2. Wash with Anti-bacterial soap the night before and the morning of your surgery.

3. Leave your valuables at home or give them to a family member for safe keeping.

4. Following completion of the surgical procedure, the athlete will remain in the recovery room until awake and vital signs are stable (usually one hours). The patient is then taken to one day surgery for usually one hour and then released.

5. Unless otherwise discussed, an athletic trainer will meet you and transport you to the surgery location and pick you up when finished.

6. If a change in physical status develops, such as cold, persistent cough, fever, skin rash or important change in condition for which you are to have surgery, notify your surgeon, or the athletic trainer (phone numbers above).

7. Wear loose fitting clothing the day of surgery.

Arrival time & date: _____   Surgery time:_____

Other Instructions:

08/11/03

Konin JG, Frederick MA. *Documentation for Athletic Training.* Thorofare, NJ: SLACK Incorporated; 2005.

James Madison University Sports Medicine

Staff Professional Goals and Achievements

Name: _____ Year: _____

Goal # 1: _____

Plan To Obtain Goal:

Resources Necessary:

Justification:

Date Goal Met:	Goal Not Met
Reason Goal Not Met:	

Goal # 2: _____

Plan To Obtain Goal:

Resources Necessary:

Justification:

Date Goal Met:	Goal Not Met
Reason Goal Not Met:	

_____	_____	_____	_____
Director of Sports Medicine	Date	Staff Signature	Date

Konin JG, Frederick MA. *Documentation for Athletic Training.* Thorofare, NJ: SLACK Incorporated; 2005.

JONES UNIVERSITY SPORTS MEDICINE CENTER
PHYSICIAN REFERRAL FORM

Date:_____   File#_____

To: _____(Physician's Name)
       _____ is a member of Jones University's
       _____team. He/She has been seen in the Sports Medicine Center for the following condition:
       _____

****
BUSINESS MANAGER:

_____   Attached you will find personal insurance information covering this athlete. Please file with the
          personal insurance company. The Athletic Department will pay that portion of the charges not paid by the
          personal Insurance.

_____   Please send a copy of the charges to the Athletic Department for payment. This athlete has no personal
          insurance to cover these charges. The Athletic Department will make payment. *

_____   Please file with the athlete's personal insurance and send the remaining charges to the Athletic Department.
          The Athletic Department will forward them to the athlete's parents for payment. (This illness/injury was
          not related to participate in the Athletic Program.) *

_____   Please send a copy of the charges to the Athletic Department. The Athletic Department will forward them
          to the parents for payment. The parents have no insurance to cover this athlete. (This illness/injury was not
          related to participation in the Athletic Program.) *
****

You are hereby authorized to release to the Athletic Trainer of Jones University any and all information regarding
my condition when under treatment or observation by you.

_____(Athlete's Signature)   _____ Date
****

To be completed by physician:

Finding/Diagnosis_____
          Recommendations/Instructions/To Patient/To Athletic Trainer:
_____
_____
_____
_____
_____
_____

_____ Physician's Signature   _____ Date
****
Please send a copy of this form and billing statements to:
Head Athletic Trainer, ATC, Jones University Box 1674, Smithville, LA 70402
****
The Jones University Athletic Department appreciated your cooperation and help in the care of our athletes. Thank
You.

Konin JG, Frederick MA. *Documentation for Athletic Training*. Thorofare, NJ: SLACK Incorporated; 2005.

MEDICAL PROCEDURES

If ill at home or unable to attend practice or scheduled contest, call coach, athletic trainer, or leave a message.

If taken ill on campus, notify coach, coach's offices, athletic trainer or Student Health Services.

If injured during practice or game, follow the instructions of the doctor or athletic trainer.

If injured and confined in dorm, report to coach and athletic trainer as requested.

All athletes who are injured or ill and cannot compete will be placed on the disabled list by the athletic trainer. Anyone not on this list is expected to report to practice and games.

If the services of a physician are needed, the student-athlete will be referred to by either or the athletic trainer or Student Health Services.

The student-athlete will be required to report at designated times for treatment or consultation.

The student-athlete may be returned to the active list on the advice of the team physician or athletic trainer.

Accurate and complete records on each student-athlete will be kept in Student Health Services, the physician's or athletic trainer's office.

Every student-athlete on every team is covered by insurance for any injury incurred in organized practice or game or when traveling from organized practice or game. The Athletics Department will try to get cooperation of your parents and their accident and health policies whenever possible.

The Athletics Department is NOT responsible for any bill incurred by a student-athlete who _sees_ a physician, has X-rays, or other treatment without the knowledge or permission of the team physician or athletic trainer.

Injury or illness unrelated to intercollegiate athletics participation are not the responsibility of the Athletics Department.

_____   _____
Athlete's Name Print   Athlete's Signature

_____   _____
Date   Social Security Number

Catastrophic Injury Incident Report

Name of Injured: _____Age:_____

Date and Time of Injury:_____

Nature of Injury: _____

Location of Injury:_____

Weather at Time of Incident: _____

External/Environmental Factors: _____

Brief Description of Incident: _____

_____

_____

_____

_____

_____

_____

_____

_____

_____

_____

Action Taken: _____

_____

_____

_____

_____

_____

_____

_____

_____

Name of Person Reporting Incident: _____

Signature of Person Reporting Incident: _____Date:_____

Department Supervisor:_____

Signature of Department Supervisor:_____Date:_____

INDEX

WAIT

...There's More!

SLACK Incorporated's Professional Book Division offers a wide selection of products in the field of Athletic Training. We are dedicated to providing important works that educate, inform and improve the knowledge of our customers. Don't miss out on our other informative titles that will enhance your collection.

Special Tests for Orthopedic Examination, Second Edition
Jeff G. Konin, PhD, AT, PT; Denise Wiksten, PhD, ATC; Jerome A. Isear, Jr., MS, PT, ATC-L; and Holly Brader, MPH, ATC, CHES
352 pp., Soft Cover, 2002,
ISBN 1-55642-591-0, Order #45910, **$36.95**

This concise manual is a valuable reference for identifying and performing special tests used during an orthopedic examination. Now available in a spiral-bound format-perfect for the reader to lay-flat and refer to as they are practicing the tests. Students, clinicians, and rehabilitation professionals will enhance their ability to interpret and evaluate their findings.

Reimbursement for Athletic Trainers
Marjorie Albohm, MS, ATC/L; Dan Campbell, PT, ATC; and Jeff G. Konin, PhD, AT, PT
176 pp., Soft Cover, 2001,
ISBN 1-55642-408-6, Order #44086, **$37.95**

Reimbursement for Athletic Trainers is the first comprehensive publication tracing the history of the NATA reimbursement initiative and outlining the specific processes of obtaining reimbursement for athletic trainers. This innovative text is organized in a "how-to" approach to filing claims, appealing denials, and approaching payers. Reimbursement in all practice settings is explored.

Practical Kinesiology for the Physical Therapist Assistant
Jeff G. Konin, PhD, AT, PT
240 pp., Soft Cover, 1999,
ISBN 1-55642-299-7, Order #42997, **$38.95**

Quick Reference Dictionary for Athletic Training
Julie N. Bernier, EdD, ATC
384 pp., Soft Cover, 2002,
ISBN 1-55642-461-2, Order #44612, **$28.95**

Principles of Pharmacology for Athletic Trainers
Joel Houglum, PhD; Gary Harrelson, EdD, ATC; and Deidre Leaver-Dunn, PhD, ATC
440 pp., Hard Cover, 2005,
ISBN 1-55642-594-5, Order #45945, **$44.95**

Athletic Training in Occupational Settings
Susan Finkam, MS, ATC, LAT, CEA
168 pp., Soft Cover, 2004,
ISBN 1-55642-632-1, Order #46321, **$37.95**

Athletic Training Exam Review: A Student Guide to Success, Second Edition
Lynn Van Ost, RN, PT, ATC, MEd; Karen Manfre, ATR, MA; and Karen Lew, MEd, ATC, LAT
240 pp., Soft Cover, 2003,
ISBN 1-55642-638-0, Order #46380, **$36.95**

Practical Exam Preparation Guide of Clinical Skills for Athletic Training
Herb Amato, DA, ATC; Christy Venable Hawkins, MS, ATC; and Steven L. Cole, MEd, ATC, CSCS
336 pp., Soft Cover, 2002,
ISBN 1-55642-572-4, Order #45724, **$27.95**

Clinical Pathology for Athletic Trainers: Recognizing Systemic Disease
Dan O'Connor, MS, PT, ATC
288 pp., Soft Cover, 2001,
ISBN 1-55642-469-8, Order #44698, **$36.95**

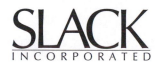